Beauty without the Scalpel

Medical Face and Body Modifications without Surgery

Carlos Soria, M.D., Ph.D.

LCCN 2012937570

ISBN 978-0-9852459-0-0

Cover Design by Jason Crye

Published by Villa of Youth Publications
P.O. Box 433856
San Diego, CA 92143
www.villaofyouth.com
619-892-2157
888-901-2744

and

Penny Callmeyer
Tiger Lilly Enterprises
P. O. Box 41325
Sacramento, CA 95841
office: 916-692-5054
http://pennycallmeyer.com
http://tigerlilly.us

Printed by Color House Graphics, Grand Rapids, Michigan

Dedication

Knowledge is not the invention of a few but rather the collective summary of endless numbers of dedicated men and women in the medical arts. They have contributed their experience and knowledge to provide procedures for those not only seeking to "feel good" but to also "look good." While painters use a canvas, sculptors work with clay, we aesthetic doctors use the body and face as our pallet. So, by simple logic this book is dedicated to those thousands of patients who are gracious enough to lend us their faces and bodies in order to allow us to practice and improve the Art of Non-Surgical Medical and Aesthetic Modifications.

Contents

Foreword

In today's world, "looking good" is as important as "feeling good." The reason is simple: whether you are looking for a job, competing in a social setting, or seeking a prospective spouse, people are drawn to attractive people. If you take pride in your appearance, people will be drawn to you, and this gives you the opportunity to show them your inner beauty as well. This also encompasses your figure, hairdo, clothing, posture, body language and even how white your teeth are! It is human nature to want to be surrounded by attractive, positive people. It takes work and time to put your best foot forward, but in the long run, you will have more success and will find doors opening for you if you present a positive self image.

This book is intended to help educate you in the procedures that are available in your quest for physical beauty. We will discuss what you need to know to determine balance, harmony, projection, mass, and horizontal/vertical proportions so that you may determine what your needs will be for optimum aesthetic beauty. We share vital information to educate you in procedures such as peels, soft tissue fillers, anti-gravitational threads, Botox and more, so that when you visit an aesthetic physician you can speak intelligently and confidently so as to make the wisest decisions. The more you educate yourself, the more wisely you can communicate with your doctor. Don't be like some celebrities who find themselves on the "worst cosmetic procedure of the year" list!

It took me 35+ years of professional practice and working with many patients to really understand beauty and how to modify anatomical structures in order to satisfy people who for one reason or another were not to happy with what they saw in the mirror.

As an example: one patient who attracted my attention was a 92 year old woman who came to me for a consultation. She complained that she had been unhappy with the size of her nose her entire life. She came from a very conservative family that was against any type of plastic surgery. When she married, her husband was of the same school, therefore she continued to look into the mirror everyday at her dreaded nose. Eventually her husband had passed and her children where busy with their own lives. By this time, she was 75 years of age and was still unhappy with the image in the mirror. It took her more than 17 years to finally opt for corrective surgery. Now she has the self-esteem she had longed for, even at her age. It was important to her that when she was laid to rest, people would look at her and not her nose.

This book is a guideline for those patients who wish to change or improve any part of their body. You can do it! Modern medical aesthetic procedures allow us to reshape you without the use of the scalpel to achieve the "look" that is so important to you.

Keep one thing in mind...Beauty is in the eye of the beholder. Please understand and accept that changing the way you look is not going to make you a better person, or help you to recapture the love you lost or even be more popular. No! Improving the way you look is just as important as improving your knowledge, your manners, or even your clothing. They are all a way to pave "the road to happiness and a more successful life."

What I want you to achieve is a better understanding of how with modern technology you can go a long way to improving your face and body without the use of the scalpel !

Introduction

I am sure that when you saw the title *Beauty without the Scalpel,* you reacted saying, "what an exaggeration!" And you are right, but, you see, the title was chosen to call your attention to the "new direction" the medical industry is moving toward. Americans of the new generation (age 35-55) do not want their bodies or faces to be submitted to a scalpel, the anesthesiologist, the operating room, a few days of hospitalization, a long recuperation at home, substantial expense, and the possible risks of a surgical procedure that is not successful. They're not interested in a "no guarantee" surgery that, in some cases, requires another "revision" procedure (with subsequent risk, expense, and time).

The information you will find in this book is intended to give you, the patient, enough knowledge (at least at a basic level) to be able to evaluate your aesthetic needs and to know as well the different types of "noninvasive" medical procedures available, in order to make an educated decision as to how to improve your face or your body.

Ultimately, the information provided will help you be prepared when you are in front of the aesthetic physician. You will not only understand his or her explanations but you will be in a position to ask important questions about the techniques or procedures your doctor is offering. Of course, the best recommendation is for you to go to a "Board Certified Specialist." Though that is the ideal, the reality is that there are nonmedical providers from other specialties that are becoming "aesthetic doctors" and after a "weekend" seminar they want to "treat" your face. The reason is simple, our new generations are becoming aware of how they look and that the face and body have a "market value." An attractive appearance may promote higher self-esteem, a better job, a better social position, and perhaps a more desirable partner.

In the event that you do not have the time or money for a procedure at this time, at least you will have done your homework and will know what your options are if and when you decide to take these measures in the future.

Ask yourself the followings questions:

1. Do you believe that changing or altering a part of your face or body could bring you better future opportunities?
2. Would you prefer to have these improvements without a surgical procedure?
3. Are you concerned, after hearing reports, that the use of anesthesiology has risks, that some patients have experienced problems from cardiorespiratory issues to sudden death? The statistics can be frightening.
4. Are you concerned about being treated in a conventional hospital because frequently bacterium resistant to most antibiotics live in the operating rooms and beds? (Two years ago I went to a general hospital for a prostate resection and as a side effect I had a bacterial infection that cost me two extra surgeries and six months in bed; I almost died from friendly fire.)
5. Are you in a financial position to pay for plastic surgeons, sterile operating rooms, an anesthesiologist, surgical assistants, instruments, surgical materials, and many "extras"?
6. Do you have enough time for a long recuperation period (hopefully without complications), time in which you may not be able to work?

7. Do you have any health issues that would prevent you from being able to take at least one week of analgesics, anti-inflammatories, muscle relaxers, or antibiotics?
8. Are you aware that after any surgery there are always "scars"? No matter how well your surgeon tries to "hide" the scars, they will always be present. There is also the possibility of hypertrophic scarring or keloids.
9. Do you know that after facial surgery there is always "numbness" of the areas next to the incisions? This is due to the severance of small nerves, which take six to twelve months to self-repair.
10. Will you have the funds to pay for another corrective procedure, again, with no guaranteed results?

If your answer to all these questions is "no," please continue reading.

If, after carefully analyzing all these questions, you come to the conclusion that plastic surgery is not for you, I want you to know that there are other alternatives.

1. Less invasive
2. Less expensive
3. Faster recuperation
4. Provable better aesthetic results.

If that sounds appealing . . .

This book is for you!

Warning: "In every medical procedure,
there are risks and side effects."

The doctor that tells you otherwise or tells you that he or she has never had a "bad result" is questionable. *"Only a doctor who does not practice does not have side effects or complications."*

Now, if you go to a nonmedical person, beauty salon, or low-cost clinic because the procedures are very economical, remember that "an economical procedure may end up being an expensive one."

Advice: Once in front of your treating physician do not forget to find out.

1. Is a medical license prominently displayed?
2. Is this procedure what the doctor specializes in?
3. Is the physician Board Certified?
4. How many seminars or conferences has he or she attended nationally and abroad?
5. How many patients have they treated in the practice? Can they prove it?
6. How many patients have suffered complications?
7. In case of a complication, who is going to take care of it? And who is going to pay for it?
8. Does the business carry medical malpractice insurance?

Finally, although this may sound harsh, you should ask: How many patients have died during your professional career? Also, how many legal situations have you encountered due to your medical work?

If you notice that your physician starts "getting nervous" or does not want to give you the information or a copy of his or her "curriculum vitae,"

Please look for another physician and clinic!

Besides all those personal questions/concerns, you must use "common sense" and observe to find answers to basic questions like these:

1. Where is the location of the consulting room or clinic?
2. Are the furnishings aesthetically pleasing?
3. Overall, is the office well maintained?

4. Are the secretary, nurse, and assistant well dressed, clean, and professional?
5. Did they schedule an appointment and see you on time?
6. Did they request your clinical history and check your vital signs (pulse, temperature, blood pressure, etc.)?
7. Were you interviewed by a physician with a professional attitude? Was he/she wearing a clean white coat and, in general, appearing to have good hygiene?
8. Were you given enough time to have all of your questions answered during your consultation?
9. Were the specific areas of treatment discussed/examined? Were photographs taken? Were you provided with an acceptable and thorough plan of treatment?
10. Were you provided a thorough and complete list of costs?
11. Were you shown the room in which the treatment will take place?
12. Were you questioned about your medical history and how any conditions could interfere with your procedure, for example, if you have diabetes or high blood pressure, could this contraindicate this procedure?
13. Were you shown before and after clinical photographs of patients with similar procedures and skin types?
14. Did the provider "guarantee," if not in a written form at least in front of his or her assistant or someone accompanying you, that your results are going to be much better?
15. Finally, at the end of your consultation were you happy not only with the doctor but with all the surroundings?

If for any reason you were left with "doubts," please don't make a quick decision that will lead to future unhappiness! *Wait!* Ask for another consultation or second opinion.

Fortunately, most consultations are "free." Take the time to arrange for that second opinion until you are confident of your choices.

Just as the doctor could find, after the interview, that you are not a good case for him, you may find that he or she is not the right doctor for you. It is okay to say no, as long as it is done with courtesy and compassion.

In order for you to be well informed when you go for your "consultation," you need to read this book carefully and thoroughly, so your doctor will know that you are not a typical "layperson." On the contrary, you will be able to interact with the doctor intelligently and be well-informed about the options.

Even more, after reading this book you will be able to tell the doctor precisely what you want. For example, if your skin is dark and tends to hyperpigment, you will not ask the doctor for a peel. You will know that if you have keloids, you cannot have surgery on the face (unless it is an emergency).

In another example, if you want lip augmentations, you must know the different types of materials to use, the quality, the price, and the duration of the effects. Many times the patient's desire to be treated is such that he or she easily becomes the prey of charlatans.

Just to give you an example, the following ad appeared in our daily newspaper:

"Butt Augmentation"
No surgery, instant results, permanent
$500.00
Telephone in Mexico 01152-664-XXXX

Regularly when we use soft tissue fillers, the cost of the procedure is 50 percent materials and 50 percent the doctor's fee.

If the person in this ad uses an average of 350 c.c. per cheek, that means a total of 700 c.c. is needed for the procedure. Let's say from the $500 the patient pays, $250 goes for the material. If we divide a 700 c.c. bottle into $250, the cost per c.c. is $0.33/ c.c..

What kind of material can they inject at a cost of $.33/c.c. when in the American market the least expensive is Vitresil 1000 (Richard James Inc.) at $10 per c.c.? If we multiply, the cost is $7,000, plus another $7,000 for the doctor. The final cost of the procedure would be $14,000. How can this procedure be done for $500?

Now you know that you have to ask what kind of product is being injected, and where does it come from?

Another example: a vial of Botox (Allergan) costs the doctor $400. With that bottle, the doctor can inject three patients, delivering thirty-three units per patient (the bottle has 100 units). If the doctor charges $400 per patient, his or her profit is 200 percent, because the first patient "pays for the bottle." So when you are offered a "cheap Botox treatment," you will have to ask: How many units are you getting and how fresh is the bottle? You should know that once the Botox is activated, its effects might last only four hours.

Do you see how useful it is to know basic information so you will not be taken for a ride?

Chapter 1
Basic Procedural Steps

Anatomy and Physiology

To start, the skin is an organ that weighs approximately six pounds. Its basic function is to serve as a protective shield that isolates our internal universe from the surrounding outside environment.

Acting as our "presentation card" to others, the skin also helps to maintain the body temperature and transmits sensorial information. Finally, the skin protects us from bacteria and other aggressors.

The skin is divided into layers:

1. The "Epidermis" is formed by the most superficial exterior cells, which "shed" or exfoliate every two weeks. Once they become superficial, they die just like the leaves of a tree and they fall off.
2. The "Dermis" or second layer (underneath the epidermis) predominately has an abundance of collagen

and elastic fibers that provide a strong support structure. The stronger this support, the less "sagging" of the skin in middle-age patients. The sun is the number one enemy. U.V. damage needs to be avoided. Nowadays, many treatments are geared to "strengthen" or "reinforce" or "regenerate" this important structure.

3. The third structure, underneath the dermis, is made of subcutaneous cellular tissue, abundant fat cells in charge of storing calories, in unlimited amounts.

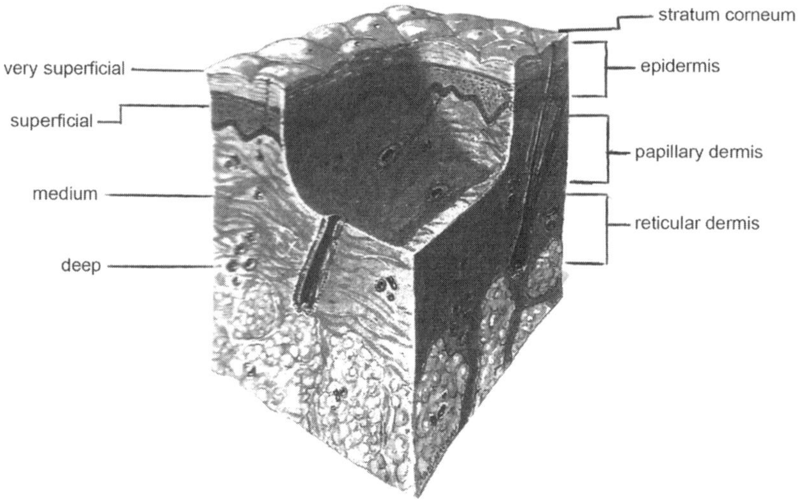

Layers of the skin

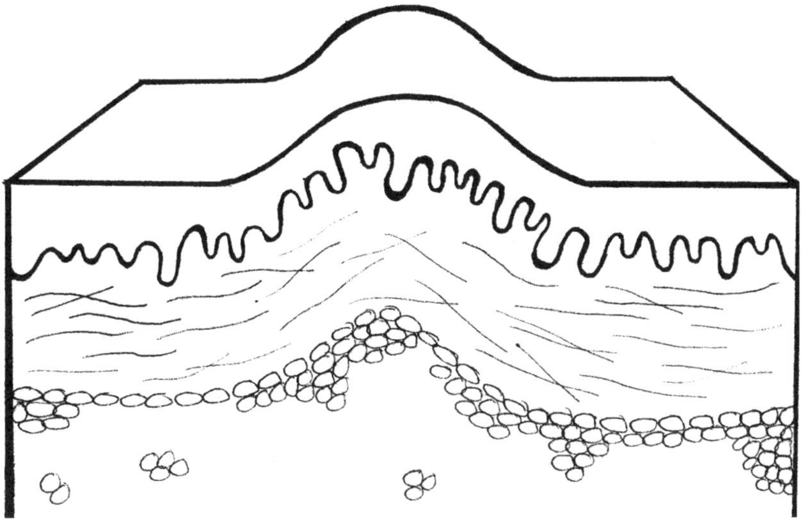

A skin fold

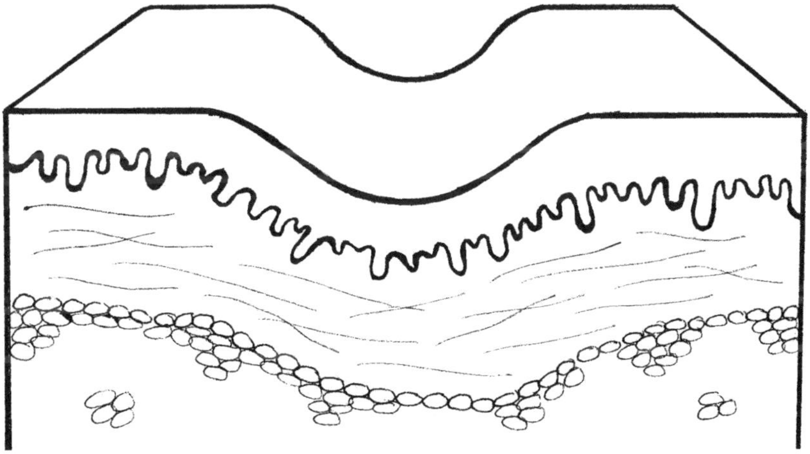

A skin furrow

How Food Intake Impacts Skin

Remember, only 1,500 calories a day are needed; more than that goes into storage for a "rainy day." The tragedy of our generation is that since our food was "industrialized," it became junk food, and junk goes to the trunk (and everywhere else). We humans tend to eat what we like and not what we need.

The international example is the fast food restaurants; the billboard says "over 99 billion served," but it doesn't say how many people have died just to have a few moments of gratification or how many people are suffering from diabetes, hypertension, or obesity.

Can you imagine how many hours and years are lost due to incapacity or pain, due to degenerative diseases produced by this junk food?

If we talk about fat, we must mention the "lethargic" effect of thousands and thousands of calories produced by beer. It is easy to conclude that beer is sold in "six packs" because statistics say that the average consumption of an American is six beers at a time, beer that is consumed accompanied by snacks, pizza, and other junk food, while watching football and sitting as far away as possible from the gym equipment.

What about our lovely children? Will they go to school and drink sodas and eat junk food?

If you are responsible for purchasing the food at the supermarket, you should purchase no more sodas. If your family is thirsty, give them water (H_2O). No more cakes, beers, ice creams; you should know by now what is not good for you. Actually, the day we become vegetarians who consume only "raw food" will be the day we become healthier!!!

Once you heat, cook, steam, or microwave food, you "denature" the proteins, that is to say that food is only good if you can eat it in its natural form. Fire (heat) destroys the nutrients and the proteins in meat. We are supposed to eat meat because it contains proteins, but oh surprise! Once you barbecue it, goodbye proteins; the same thing happens with any other food!

A suggestion: Tomorrow get rid of your stove and microwave and eat only "raw vegetables."

The worst addiction in the world is not alcohol or hard drugs. No! It is to food! The United States is number one in obesity in the world, and Mexico is number two; the United States is number two in childhood obesity, and Mexico is number one.

While we are young our skin is nice and firm. The tragedy of solar damage, the environmental toxins, the chronic poisoning of smoking, and age in general will damage the skin, breaking down the elasticity and collagen fibers. The skin will "sag" and become redundant. Atrophy sets into the subcutaneous fat cell deposits, and one day, especially after a heavy drinking night, we wake up, go to the bathroom, look in the mirror, and think "What is my mother/father doing in the mirror?" From that day on, nothing is the same…

What Are Wrinkles

Everything in this world tends to "oxidate," that is, to degenerate, and humans are not the exception. The skin gradually loses its dermis support and its ability to distend itself and come back to its original position. We become like Shar Pei dogs.

Appearing during the aging process, wrinkles are "redundancies" of skin that fold into the facial muscles.

For simplicity, wrinkles can be classified as

A) Fine ***B) Medium*** ***C) Deep***

Wrinkles are the most apparent clinical sign of aging of the skin; changes in wrinkles "push" many patients to their doctors.

Who would have believed that a poison, yes a poison, originated by a bacteria called Clostridium botulinum, was to become in 2012, the number one cosmetic procedure in the world?

Botox is not only used by dermatologists, but by many other types of doctors and by nonmedical people, such as in beauty salons and gymnasiums. The average cost is four hundred dollars per treatment. It is used to minimalize the facial expression, in a temporary way—yes only for three to five months—so you have to spend a minimum of twelve hundred dollars a year to maintain the effect.

Fine wrinkles are more evident in a resting position and less evident with facial expression, because those lines are diminished or eliminated when the skin is "pushed in" during smiling.

Medium lines are diminished when the face is at rest, but obvious when muscular contraction takes place as with crow's-feet.

Finally, deep wrinkles are obvious folds when the skin is at rest, for example, the depression from the nose to the corner of the mouth (nasolabials). Their presence is more accentuated with facial expressions. When we smile, the muscle shortens and pushes in the skin.

Forehead lines are produced by the contraction of the frontal muscle, crow's-feet by the eyelid orbicular muscle, and the nasolabial fold by the contraction of the elevation of the angle of the mouth and zygomatic major.

Reasons for Aging

Wouldn't it be wonderful if, as time goes by, our skin could remain nice, soft, and clean with good elasticity, just like when we were teenagers (but without the pimples)?

But no, gravity has its way and everything tends to fall; the skin is no exception.

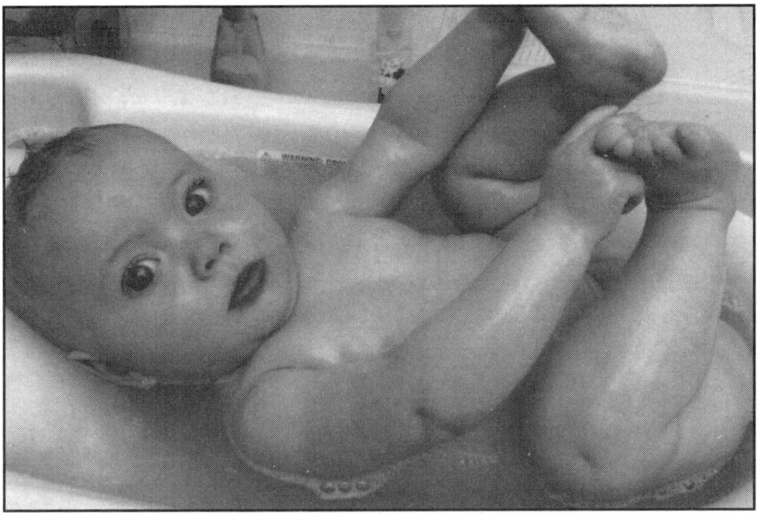

Three-month-old skin. Are you jealous?

Genetic Factors

When I asked my father how my wife would look at sixty-five years of age, he replied, "just look at her mother." Genetics are our biological inheritance, and that is a combination of our parents' genes, good and bad, and not only parents, but any other blood relative.

So if we happen to be short, and not good looking, we should find a wife who is tall and pretty (preferably with money) so our children can improve their genetic inheritance and have better odds in this discriminating society—right or wrong?

Social Factors

"We are what we eat" is a universal truth. Because the skin is not only a protective shield, but also an "excretion" organ, the skin allows the body to get rid of unwanted toxins and "waste" through perspiration.

Basically, God made us vegetarians. If meat were good for us, we could eat it directly from the dead animal (just like any other carnivore), but since men discovered "fire," the fire transforms something that is inedible to something edible (especially if we add steak sauce). We already mentioned that by placing meat on a grill we "destroy" the proteins so the meat retains no valuable nutrients.

Environmental Factors

The sun is our friend, a great benefactor, but it is our skin's worst enemy. That is because the sun emits radiation that, accumulated over the years, produces "photoaging." Our skin will reveal fine wrinkles, an increase in pigmentation, blemishes, and dysplastic changes of the epidermis. That causes areas called actinic keratosis and possibly pre-cancerous skin lesions, all those changes are more evident at middle age.

Universal Beauty

Let's face it, nobody can remain young forever, and many of us have not been genetically favored with good-looking bodies or faces. A low percentage of the general public is "model beautiful," while a few more are "good looking"; the rest go from average to ugly. That is why cosmetic medical procedures—surgical or not—could be the answer that everyone is looking for. In the "search for perfection," humanity has created "models of beauty": rounded and Rubenesque in old times and tall and thin in our times, or dependent on the geography or culture. Since time immemorial, there has been a search for facial perfection and beauty, and the search is ongoing.

Just in the United States, approximately 650,000 patients undergo aesthetic surgical procedures of different types each year.

Today there is a renewal of beauty goals created by the Greek and Romans. Besides having athletic bodies, patients are looking for more dramatic facial contours accentuated by strong noses and prominent cheekbones with well-defined jawlines and prominent chins. Their features are the favorites of today's celebrities—models, actors, actresses, and idols of movies and television. Superheroes like Superman, Batman, and Wonder Woman and actors like Marlon Brando, Gregory Peck, Charlton Heston, Kirk Douglas, Tom Cruise, and Angelina Jolie are examples of what we wish to look like.

Those facial volumes and contours exist as a result of localization, volume, and mass of the facial soft tissues and their relationship with the subjacent bone structures.

The visual impression that a person makes has a considerable "weight" in human relationships. The clothes, makeup, hair, jewelry, posture, movement, and voice timbre contribute to our ability to stimulate a positive response from those we encounter. How about that? How many details will we observe and be influenced by in our next personal or work relationship?

During your medical consultation, your doctor needs to analyze you from the front, three-quarters and lateral views. He or she will measure, take photographs, and notice the general volume of the head, the shape of the face, relative volumes of parts related to the forehead, the medium part, and finally the lower part of the face. He or she will notice curvatures, angles, and each one of the generalities and particulars of your face. Your doctor must take into consideration the concepts of anatomy, balance, symmetry, and proportions.

Actually your doctor should be not only an M.D., but a sculptor. Ask whether he or she attends art classes, paints, or sculpts.

There are several methods for obtaining the above-mentioned goals. They all have something in common—to obtain the "key of beauty."

Artistically speaking, the skin and subcutaneous fat are the "canvas" of the face; their soft distribution upon the bone produces the appearance of youth.

Anatomy of the Face

There are six basic anatomic elements in the face.

1. Sensual, well-defined, and full lips
2. Good medial and lateral inclination
3. Well-delineated eyebrows and arches, slightly elevated in the union of the medium and lateral eyebrows
4. Triangular and straight, well-proportioned nose
5. Chin with good presence
6. Jaw angle well pronounced and in ninety-degree angle

Nevertheless, the final analysis of the anatomical configuration of the volume and features that control and dominate—this is what determines a beautiful face.

In general, the face is divided into three vertical segments: upper, medium, and lower.

If the volume of the mass and the aesthetic configuration of these three units relate among themselves and relate with the magnitude of the projection of the nasal and chin prominences, this is what determines what we perceive as "aesthetic beauty."

Basic Psychology of Beauty

Let's be honest—everybody loves beauty and youth. In any period of human history, men and woman have looked for the "fountain of eternal youth" based upon the idea that beauty and youth could make them happy. Just imagine for a minute that, before the age of plastic surgery, humans needed to adapt themselves to whatever "genes" they received through heredity. Whatever their appearance—good, mediocre or poor—it had to be for the rest of their lives.

However, with the advances of medicine, mainly plastic surgery, men and women gained the ability to be free from their genetic imposition, allowing them to manufacture their own self-image.

Just imagine. Today you can create your own body and face, simply by finding professional doctors with enough knowledge, technical equipment, and aesthetic capabilities to change any part of your body (as long as you have the financial resources). Isn't it a dream come true?

In our society, millions and millions of dollars are spent every year on cosmetics, hairstyles, spas, clothes, and surgeries just to make us feel "better, prettier, and happier," that is, to improve our self-esteem.

The sad reality is that nobody stays young and good looking forever; most of us are not blessed from birth with good-looking faces and bodies. This is why those individuals that were born good looking and have taken the time to mold the temple called the body are like shining stars when they walk into a room. People admire and idolize them. Sometimes when these "super humans" happen to be "talented" in singing, dancing, acting, and so forth, people consider them "living idols" and "larger than life" as in the case of Rudolf Valentino, a film star and sex symbol of the 1920s.

We always admire what we don't have ourselves, although today we can change practically any part of our bodies, through face-lifts, liposuction, breast augmentation, nose modifications, and chin/cheek augmentation. These procedures can be easily done for a variety of reasons, but the most important seems to be to improve self-esteem.

"I look more feminine after my breast augmentation," "my clothes fit better after my liposuction," "my face looks less tired," and so on are some of the opinions of people who have chosen cosmetic plastic procedures.

It is important that you understand that the final goal of aesthetic medicine is to improve your initial physical condition and not to obtain "perfection." Even more important to bear in mind, *"There is no such thing as perfection. Even the most beautiful people in the world are not perfect."* When we see them in films or photographs, they have been submitted to many hours with makeup, hairstylists, diets, exercise, and so forth. When photographs appear in magazines, hundreds of photographs were taken in order to choose one (not to mention the use of photo editing software).

If we had the ability to see idols first thing in the morning as soon as they wake up, without makeup, they would appear much more normal.

A popular saying is, *"Beauty is in the eye of the beholder."* Generally, extreme beauty or ugliness is the first thing that our eyes see.

The perceptive aspects of body image involve mental, visual, and space mechanisms that explain why corporal images play an important positive roll in self-image. It is generally believed that patients submitting to cosmetic procedures do acquire a big improvement in self-esteem. When you look in the mirror and you are not satisfied with what you see, you may experience feelings of concern or anxiety that can severely affect your normal functioning. Plastic or aesthetic medicine has as a final goal making a stigmatized person feel like a normal one.

In the United States, there is a fundamental union between self-esteem and physical appearance that has a "market value." Several authors suggest that aesthetic surgery and exercise are motivated by the desire to fit into the beauty patterns imposed by society.

In a simple manner, we could classify patients with aesthetic needs into two groups.

The first group is people who have physical defects acquired during birth or due to accidents. The second group comprises people that wish to improve physical aspects that they do not like.

We say that the realities given to the patient are important and permanent, so it is extremely crucial that the individual has a pretty good idea of how these changes could impact their lives.

It is not a crime to want to look better or prettier. For us doctors, it is a desire that we constantly seek in our practice. However, the diagnosis of "dysmorphia," known as Body Dysmorphic Disorder, is a psychiatric condition that consists of a constant preoccupation with a "non-existent" or "hardly noticeable" physical defect, which causes severe anxiety or even fear that interferes with the patient's social life.

Further Reading

Guimaraes Le. *PatronizQ (;ao de* um *metodo computadorizado de avaliafao fotografica do perfil facial tegumentar.* (Disserta aode Mesrado). Sao Paulo, 2003, Universidade de Sao Paulo.

Boos RM. *Estudo da influencia de angulos do perfil facial feminino na preferencia de avaliadores on-line* (Disserta ao de Mestrado). Porto Alegre, 2001. Faculdade de Odontologia da Pontificia Universidade Catolica do Reio Grande do Sul.

Czarnecki ST, Nanda RS, Currier FG. Perceptions of a balanced facial profile. Amer J *Orthodont* 1993; 104(2): 108-7,

Suguino S, Ramos AL, Terada HH, Furquim LZ, Maeda L, Silvafilho OG. Analise facial, *Rev. Dental Press Ortod Ortop Max* 1996; 1)1):86-107.

Cochrane SM, Cunningham, SJ, Hunt, NP. Perceptions of facial Appearance by Orthodontists and the General Public. JCO 1997; 331 (3): 164-168.

Okuyama CC, Martins DR. Preferendia do perfil facial tegumentar, em jovens leucodermas, melanodermas e xantodermas de ambos os sexos, avaliados por ortodontistas, leigos e artistas *plasticos. Ortadon* 197; 30: 6-16.

Farkas LG, Bryson W, Klotz J. Is Photogrammetry of face reliable? *Plast Reconstr Surg* 1980; 66(1-3): 346-55.

Doczi G. HClrmonias e Propor oes na Natureza, Arte e Arquitetura. O Poder dos Limites. Sao Palo 2000. DEDALUS; Acervo FAU 20200015058.

Gil CTLA. *Estudo da proporfao aurea na arquitetura craniofacial de individuos adultos com oe/usac normal, a partir de telerradiografias exais frontais e laterais* (Tese deDoutorado). Sao Jose dos Campos.

Cabrera CAG, Cabrera Me. Ortondontia Clinica Curitiba, 1997. Ed. Produ oes Interativas.

Morres CFA, Kean MR. Natural head positiom a basic consideration in the interpretation of cephalometric radiographs. Am J *Phy Anthrop* 1958; 16:213-234.

Lopes KB. *Avaliafoes tegumentarias, esqueleticas e dentarias do perfil facial* (Disserta ao de Mestraso) Sao Paulo, 2004. Faculdade de Odontologia da Universidade de Sao Paulo.

Viazis AD. A cephalometric Analysis Based on Natural Head Position. J *Clin Orthod* 1991. 224:172-81.

Ricketts RM. Divine proportion in facial esthetics. *Clin Plast Surg* 1982; 401

Powell N, Humphreys. B. *Proportions of the Aesthetic Face.* New York, 1948. NY: Theime-Stratton Inc.

Powell N. Aesthetic evaluation of nasal contours, em cummings CW, Frederickson JM, Harket LA. et al. *Otolaryngology-Head and Neck Surgery.* 1986. St. Louis, CV Mosby.

Merrifield LL. The profile line as an aid in critically evaluating facial esthetics. Am J *Orthod* 1996; 52:804-22..

Nassif PS, Kokoska MS. Aesthetic Facial Analysis. *Facial Plastic Surgery Clinics of North America*, 1999, 7:1, 1-15.

Farkas, LG. *Anthropometric of the head and face in medicine.* New York: Elscuiez North Holland Inc. 1981. 91, 1982.

Holdaway RA. A soft-tissue cephalometric analysis and its use in orthodontic treatment planning. Part II. Am J *Orthod*, 1084; 85:279-93.

Legan HL, Burstone CJ. Soft tissue cephalometric analysis for orthognathic survery. J *Oral Surg*, 1980;38:744-51.

Scheideman GB, Bell WH, Legan HL, Finn RA, Reisch JS. Cephalometric analysis of dentofacial normals. Am J *Orthod*, 1080; ; 78)4_:404-20.

Schwartz, AM. Rontg Enostatik-rban & Schwarzenberg. Munchen, 1958. Cephalometric analysis and its use in orthodontic treatment planning. In: Suguino S, Ramos AL, Terada HH,

Furquim LZ, Maedfa L, Silfafilho OG.Analise facial. *Rev. Dental Press Orto Ortop Max* 1996; 1 (1):86-107.

Gonzales-Ulloa M, Flores ES. Senility of the face; Basic study to understand its cauuses and effects. *Plast Reconsruc Surg* 1965; 36:239.

Hinderer UT. Malar Implants to Improve Facial Proportions and Aging. In: Stark RB ed. *Plastic Surgery of the Head and Neck.* 1987 New York: Churchill Livingstone.

Furtado RI. Morfologia nasal, harmonia e propor ao applicadas a rinoplastia. *Rev Med Hosp Monte Klinikun*, 203 - Ceara 2(4) 18-26.

Powell, NB, Riley RW, Laub DR. A new approach to evaluation and surgery of the malar complex. *Ann Plast Surg*, 1988; mar 20(3):206-214.

Chapter 2
Facial Rejuvenation

The goal of facial skin rejuvenation is to produce nice soft, younger skin, dramatically softening the ravages of time—imperfections, blemishes, unwanted pigmentation. The result after treatment is skin "like a baby's bottom."

The topical medical preparations act upon primarily the epidermis and secondarily the dermis.

The acids and the new generation of lasers not only remove the epidermis, but they also can penetrate deeply enough to stimulate the reticular dermis, improving and remodeling the collagen fibers.

Although peelings can be used to treat or remove benign and pre-malignant lesions, the main indication in modern dermatology is for the removal of wrinkles in aging skin.

Your doctor, according to his or her experience and your type of skin, can recommend the proper treatment.

Chemical Peels

Chemical peels are defined as the application to the skin of different acids to produce a controlled inflammatory reaction upon the epidermis (in superficial peels) or in the dermis in the case of medium or deep peels. Subsequent to this inflammatory reaction, the skin regenerates itself with a much younger appearance.

Types of Depth in Peels

Peels could be classified as superficial, medium, and deep, depending on the "penetration" of the inflammatory reaction.

Superficial—acts upon the stratum corneum in epidermis

Medium—acts upon the epidermis and part of the papillary dermis

Deep—goes from the superficial to the medium and reticular dermis.

Here is a list of the different types of peels:

1. Superficial or light peelings
   a) Alpha-hydroxy acids
   b) CO_2 (+alcohol sulfur)
   c) Jessner's solution
   d) Resorcinol
   e) Salicylic acid
   f) TCA (Trichloroacetic acid 10 to 30%)
   g) Unna's paste (TCA + 10 to 30%)
2. Medium deep chemical peel
   a) Phenol 88%
   b) Trichloroacetic acid 35 to 50%
3. Deep chemical peel
   a) Baker-Gordon Formula (Phenol 44%) (open or closed)
   b) Clyde Litton formula (Phenol 44%) (open or closed)

Light Chemical Peels

The chemical agent used for topical application is not too acid, works efficiently, and is low risk. Light peels are used to modify signs of aging, especially the damage produced by accumulated solar light. This "photoaging" appears as fine wrinkles and hyper pigmentation changes (sunspots), solar damage and "reddish" color generators. These changes are evident in middle age (40 to 50 years).

Light topical preparations are generally products purchased over the counter and applied at home. All these products produce "superficial peels" with skin exfoliation.

1. Alpha-hydroxy acids
2. Azelaic acid
3. Fluorouracil (5-FU or f5U)
4. Salicylic acid
5. Retinol cream

The most frequently used are alpha-hydroxy acids (AHAs), glycolic, lactic, malic, citric, and tartaric acids. The clinical effects are relative to their concentrations and require at least six months of treatment. The chemical concentrations range from 5 to 20 percent. My favorite formula is a combination of lactic acid, resorcinol, and salicylic acid under the name of Jessner's Solution, this produces a very effective superficial peel.

Medium Peels

This type of peel can produce significant changes in the skin. The results are more obvious in expression lines, but the positive changes are not as long lasting as the ones achieved in phenol peels.

TCA (Trichloroacetic Acid) is the most frequently used chemical to obtain a medium deep action. The concentrations range from

25 to 35 percent and can produce an inflammatory depth that reaches the medium to deep reticular dermis. This concentration of TCA is not recommended for clinical use. Furthermore, it can damage the skin and produce scars of difficult resolution.

After treatment, patients should avoid direct exposure to the sun for six months, and they must accept that the skin will remain red and swollen during the next three to four months.

These peels are not advised for patients with hyperpigmented dark skin or very freckled skin.

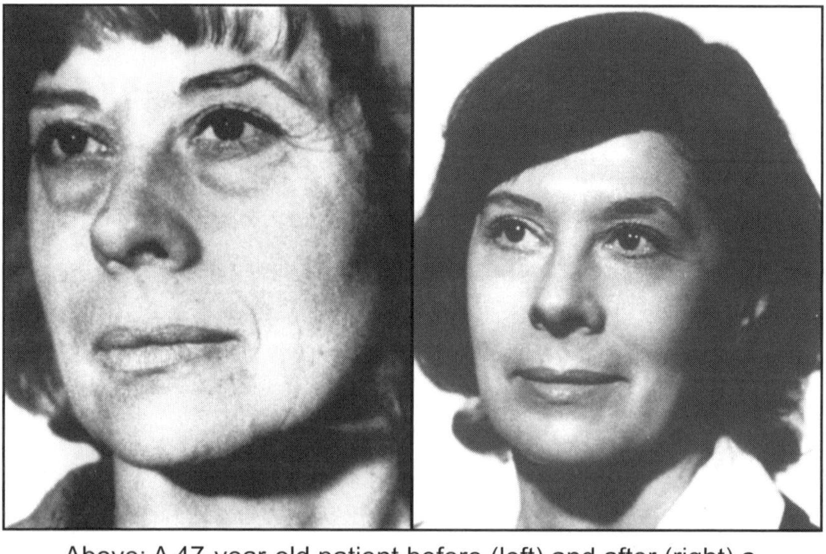

Above: A 47-year-old patient before (left) and after (right) a medium peel for the improvement of pigmentation and lesions

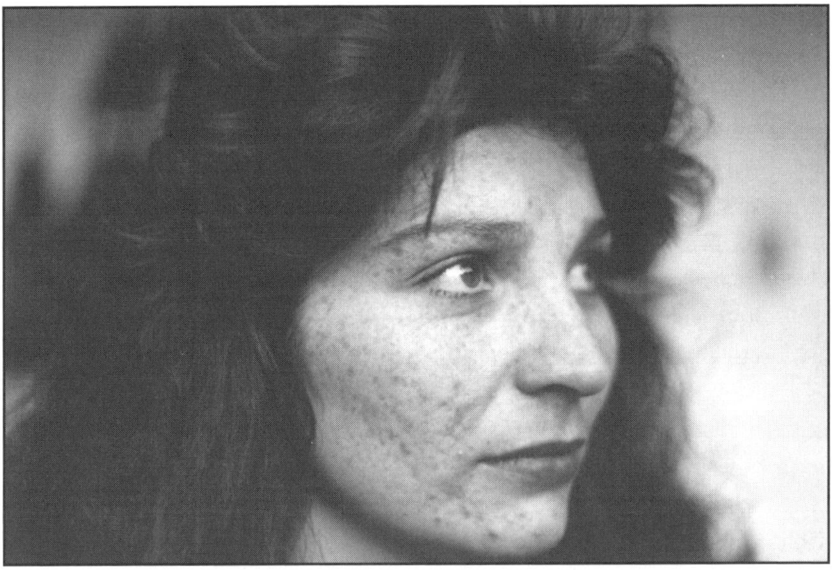

37-year old patient with acne scarring.

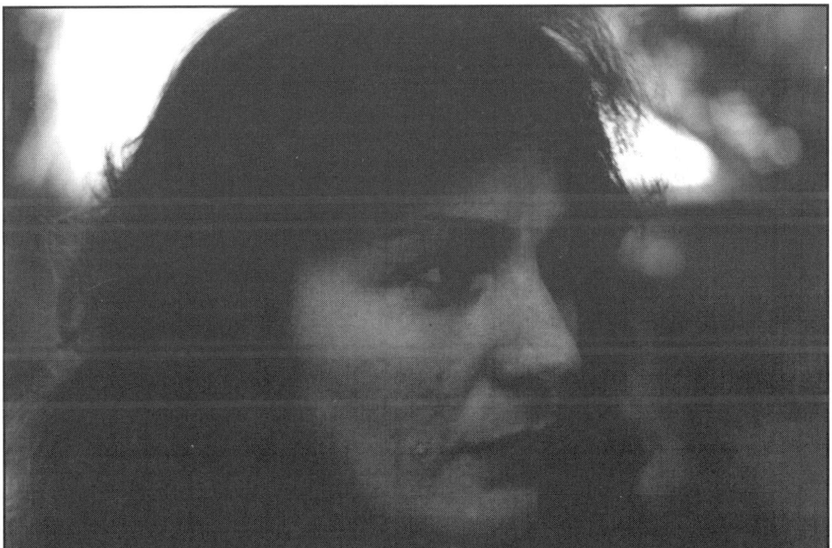

Twelve days after a medium chemical peel.

Deep Peel

By definition, deep peels produce inflammation from the surface of the skin all the way down into the deep dermis. Phenol or carbolic acid is the chosen ingredient in what we call "Baker formula." In our experience with more than ten thousand peels, we have found that this is the most successful formula, but it is also the most risky if the proper patient protocol is not followed.

Just to give you an idea, this procedure has to be performed in a well-ventilated surgical area, with intravenous sedation by an anesthesiologist, continued cardiac monitoring, and with equipment for cardiopulmonary resuscitation. It is not rare for the patient to experience "cardiac arrhythmias" or, worse, heart failure. This is not a procedure for beginning doctors, and it should be done in a hospital setting.

At those deep levels of skin, complications can be systemic or local. The local ones can be prolonged "redness" and lack of pigmentation of the skin. There are some reports of infections by bacterium or herpes, as well as scars.

Lasers

As time goes by, new technologies have provided us with CO_2 pulsation lasers, together with other variations of lasers that allow a more controlled "deep" inflammatory lesion, just as chemical peels through "ablation" (burn) of the epidermis stimulate a new generation of stronger, younger collagen.

Here the vital part is not the chemicals or the machine employed by the doctor (laser, chemical, or dermabrasion) but rather the personal experiences of the medical personnel. If your doctor feels comfortable with chemicals or a $180,000 laser, let him or her choose the technique. You as a patient are looking for the results. The professional should not "sell" you a laser or "chemical peel." No; he or she should "sell" you a result! It is like a surgeon promising to obtain better results with a "golden" scalpel rather than with a stainless steel one. You should not care about the instrument; you should only care about the results.

There are some disadvantages with lasers. For example, they cannot be applied to areas with hair like eyebrows or inside of the hairline because the hair would be destroyed. Laser produces a demarcation line between the treated and untreated area, the same way it occurs on the skin of the neck or chest. Most lasers stop at the jawline producing a noticeable demarcation line. On the other hand, chemical peels can be applied into the hairline, neck, and chest.

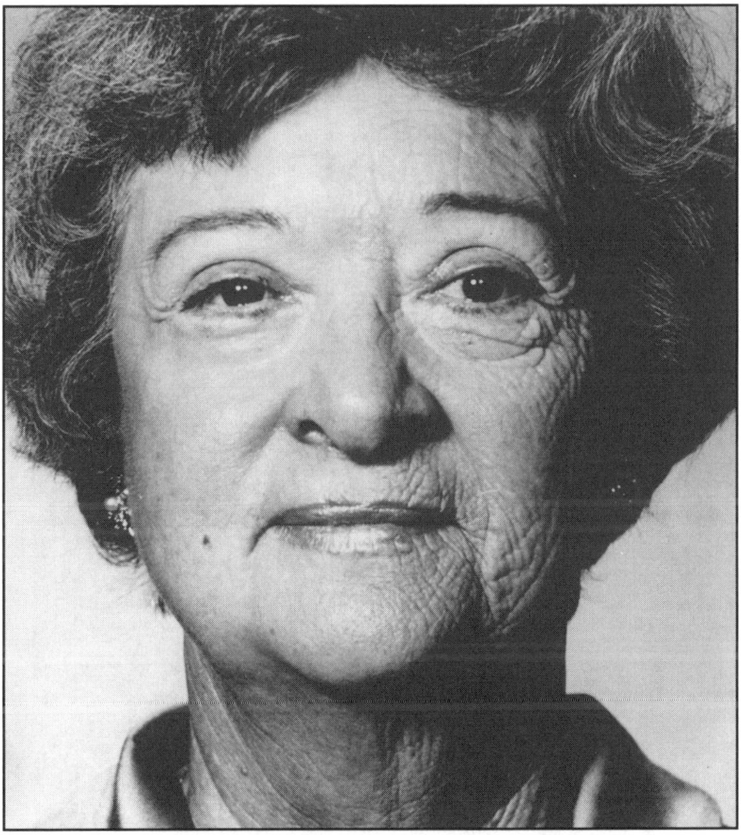

A 65-year-old patient treated with phenol on the left side of the photograph, thirty days after treatment. Note the dramatic result not only on the face but on her neck as well. (No photographic alteration)

The downside of chemical peels is that they tend to produce more "hypopigmentation" (with phenol). In our personal experience, phenol peels have a beneficial effect of more than twenty years. Remember that your doctor is the only one that should recommend a procedure, based upon his or her experience.

Results

After more than thirty-five years of practice and thousands of deep chemical peels, having compared the results with those obtained with laser CO_2, we have reached the conclusion that chemical peels are significantly better. Peels are also less expensive than using laser machines; the cost of the chemicals needed to perform a treatment is no more than one hundred dollars.

On the other hand, to perform a chemical peel takes two to three hours, and a CO_2 laser treatment takes only forty-five minutes.

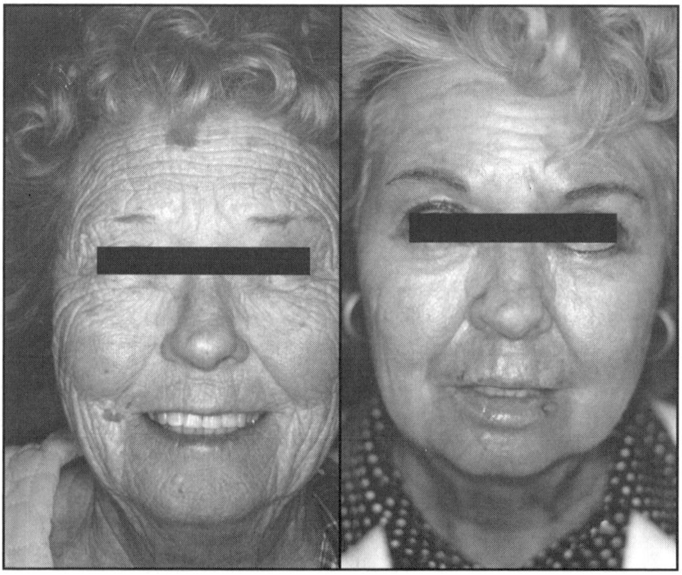

Left. 78-year-old patient with severe wrinkling
Right. Same patient twelve days after treatment with phenol.

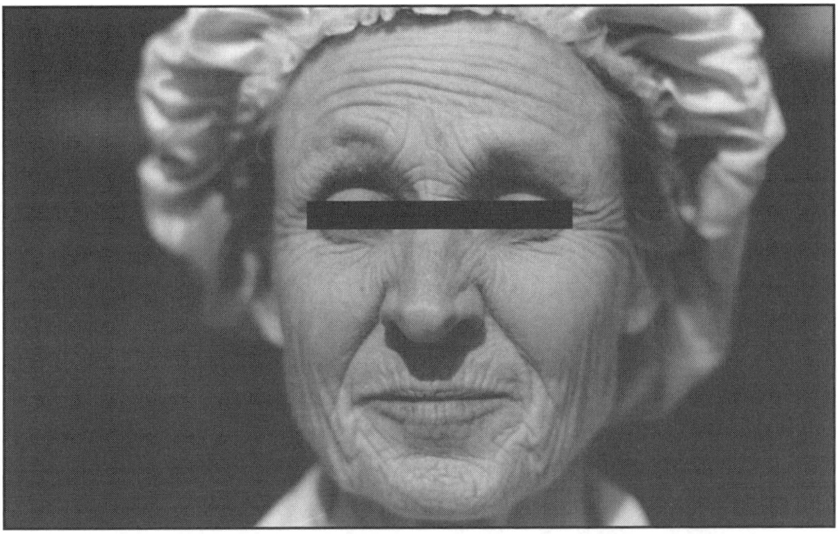

68-year-old patient before treatment

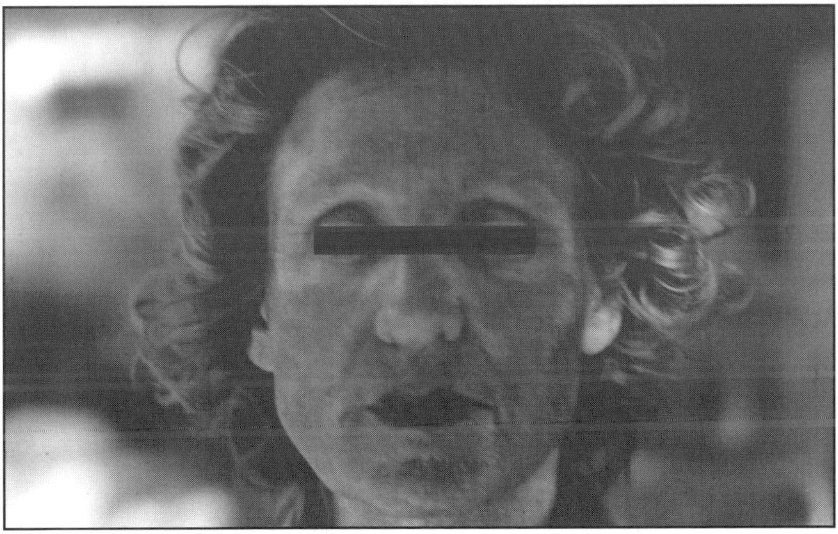

Same patient twelve days after treatment with phenol 44 percent

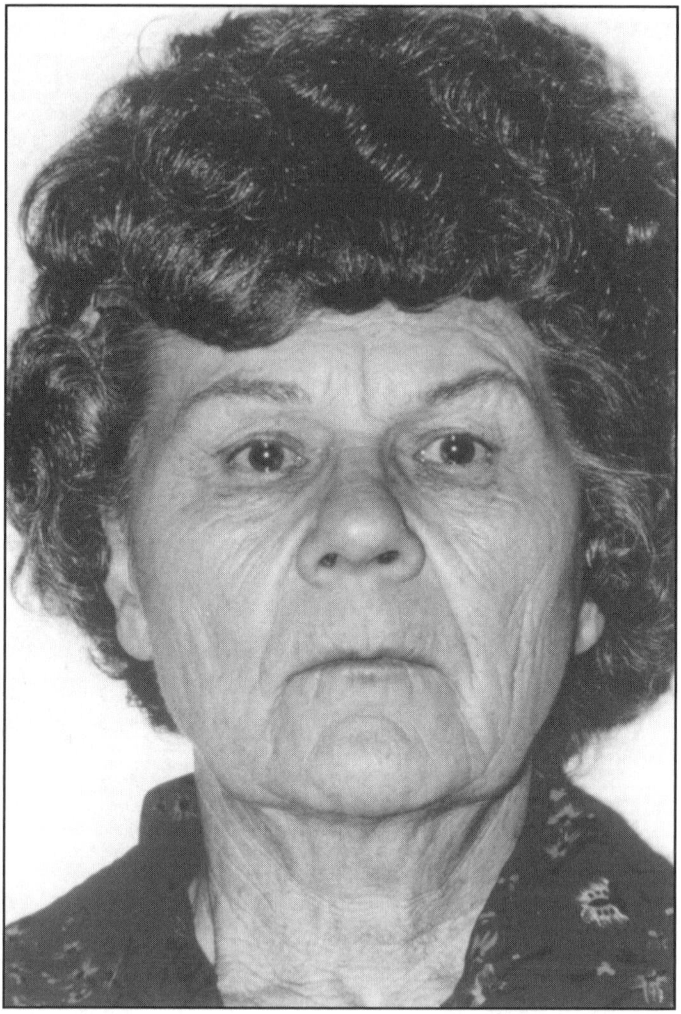

Deep skin peel: before.

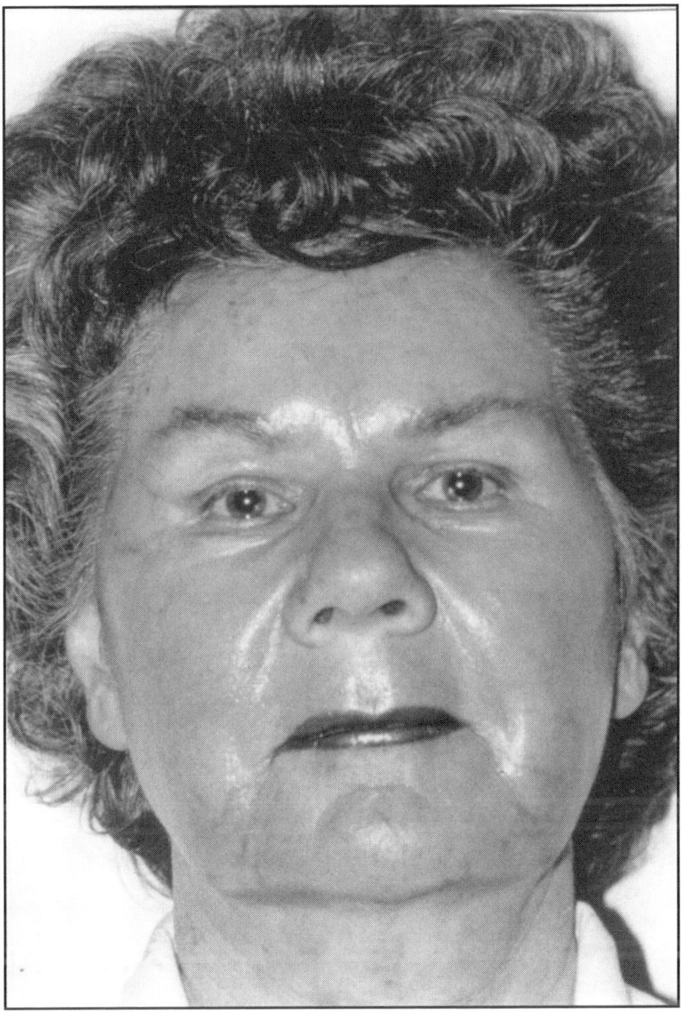

Deep skin peel: after.

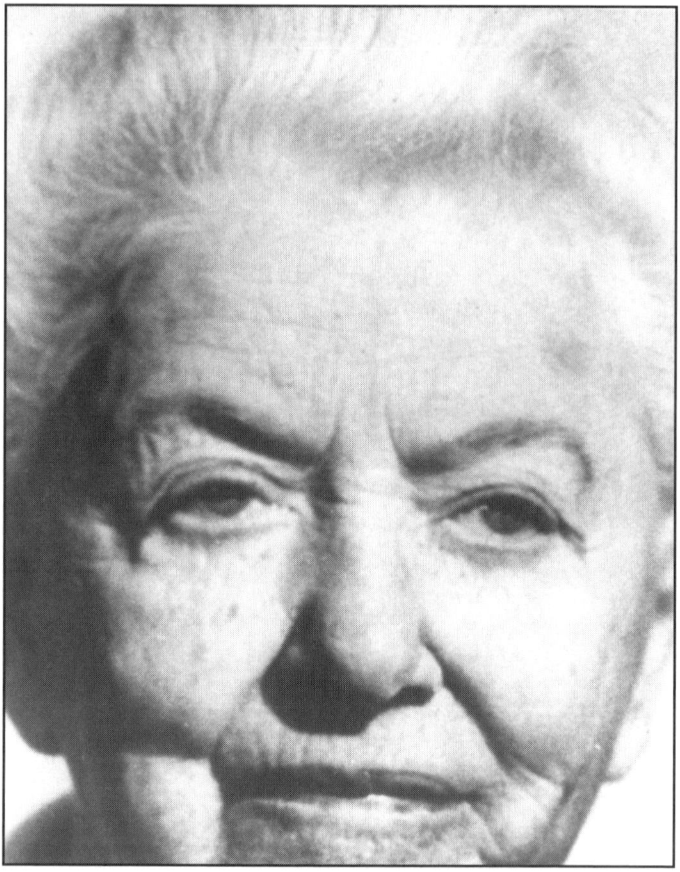

Deep skin peel: before.

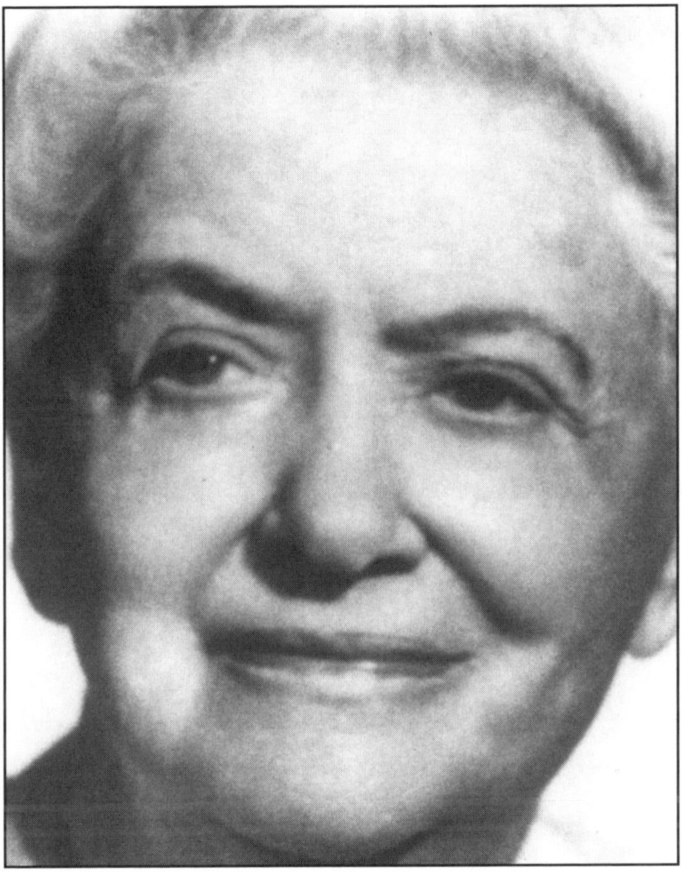

Deep skin peel: after.

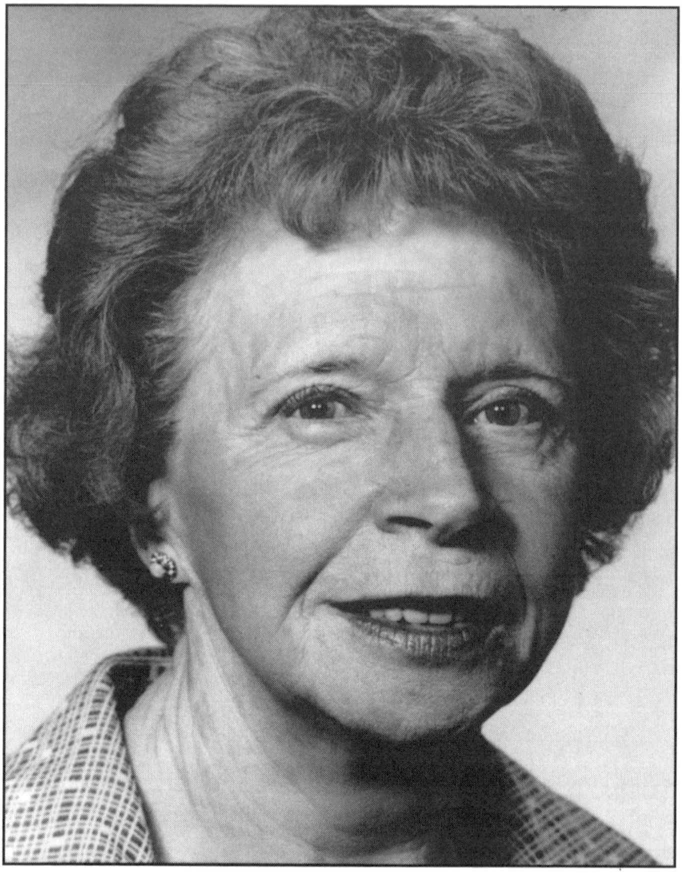

Deep skin peel: before.

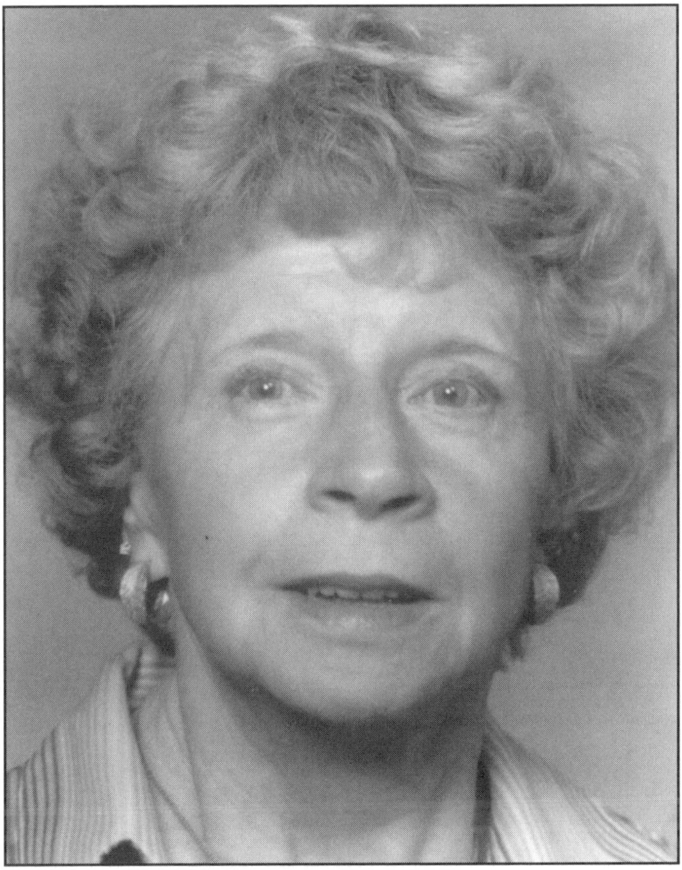

Deep skin peel: after.

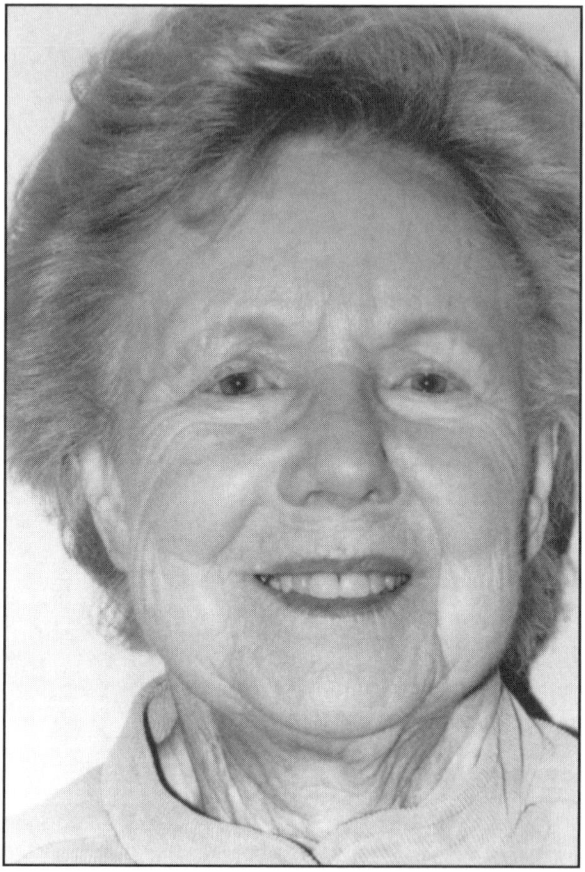

Deep skin peel: before.

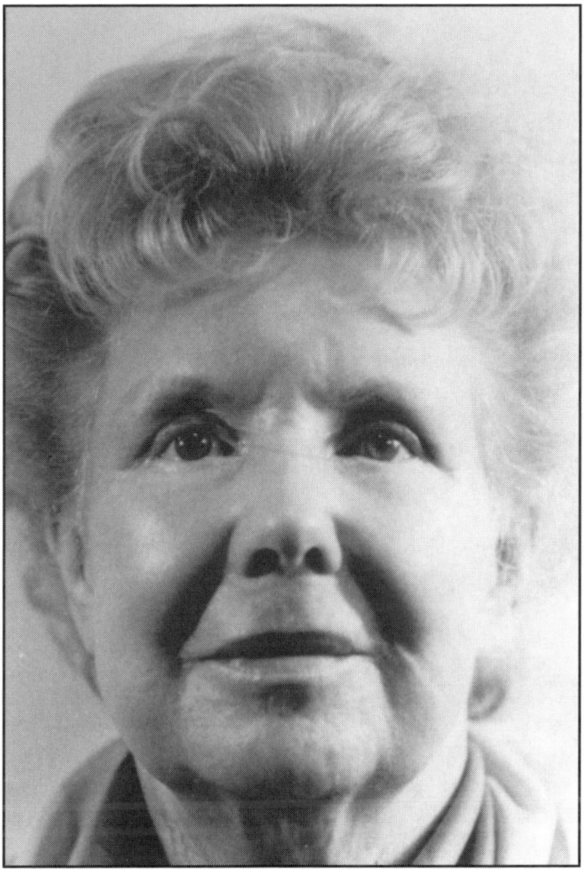

Deep skin peel: after.

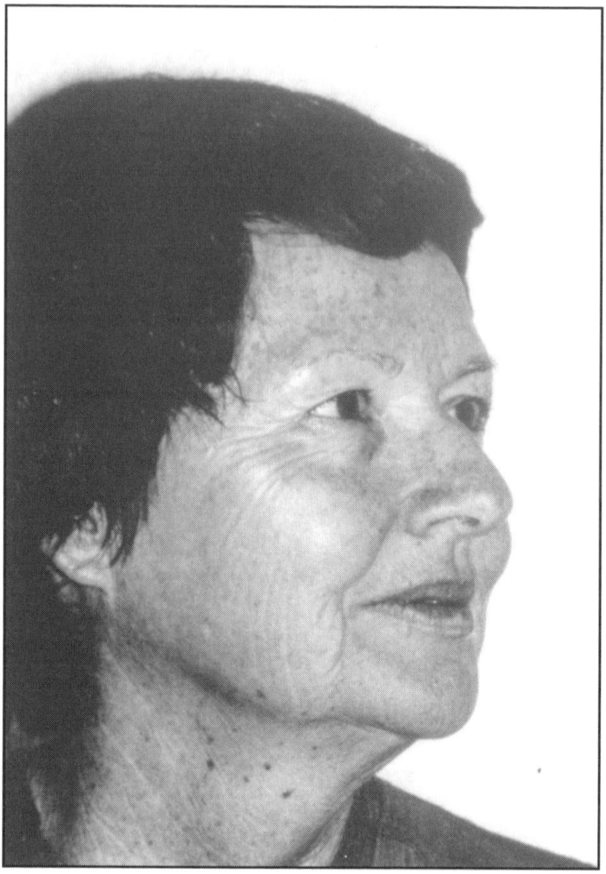

Deep skin rejuvenation: before.

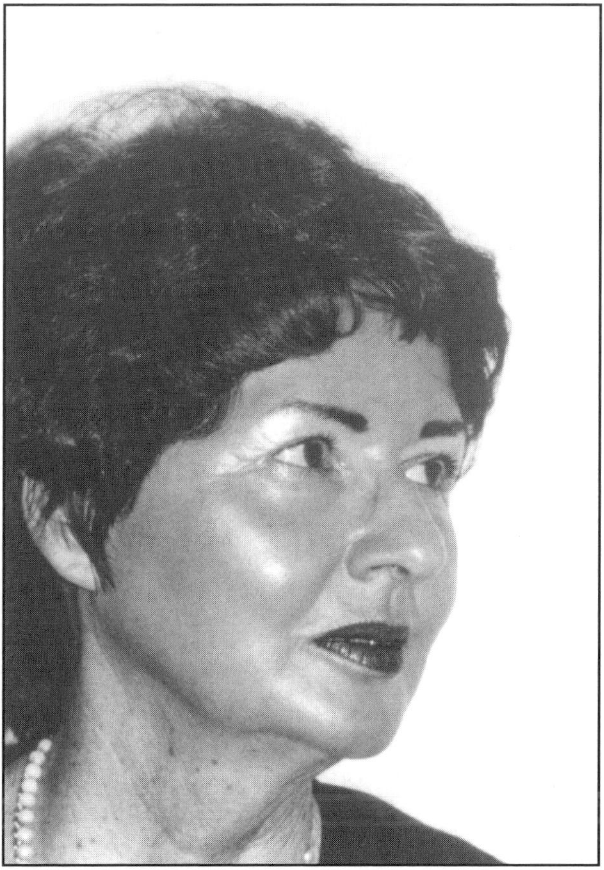

Deep skin rejuvenation: after.

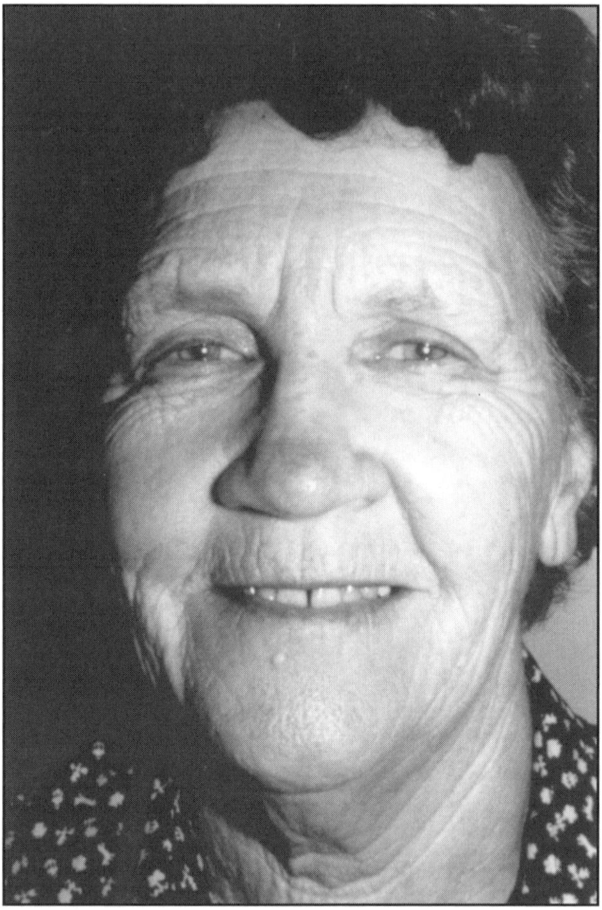

Deep skin rejuvenation: before.

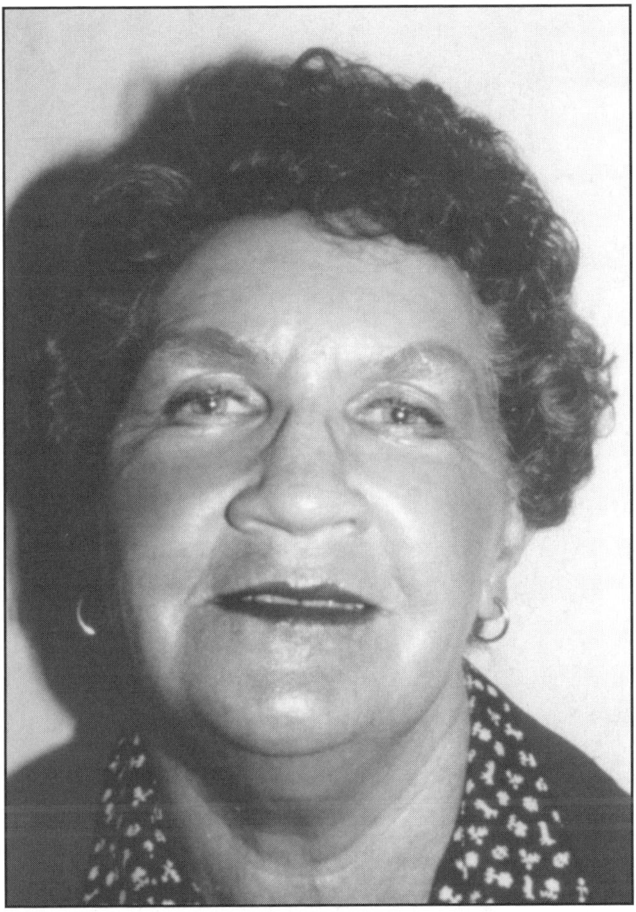

Deep skin rejuvenation: after.

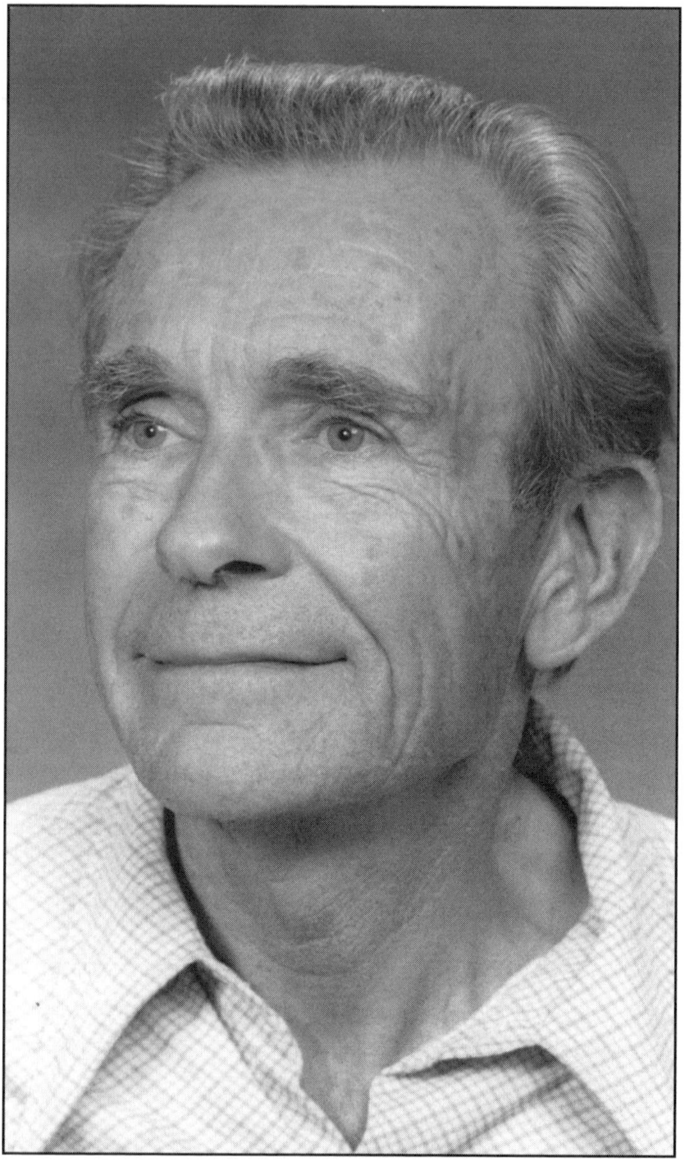

Deep skin rejuvenation: before.

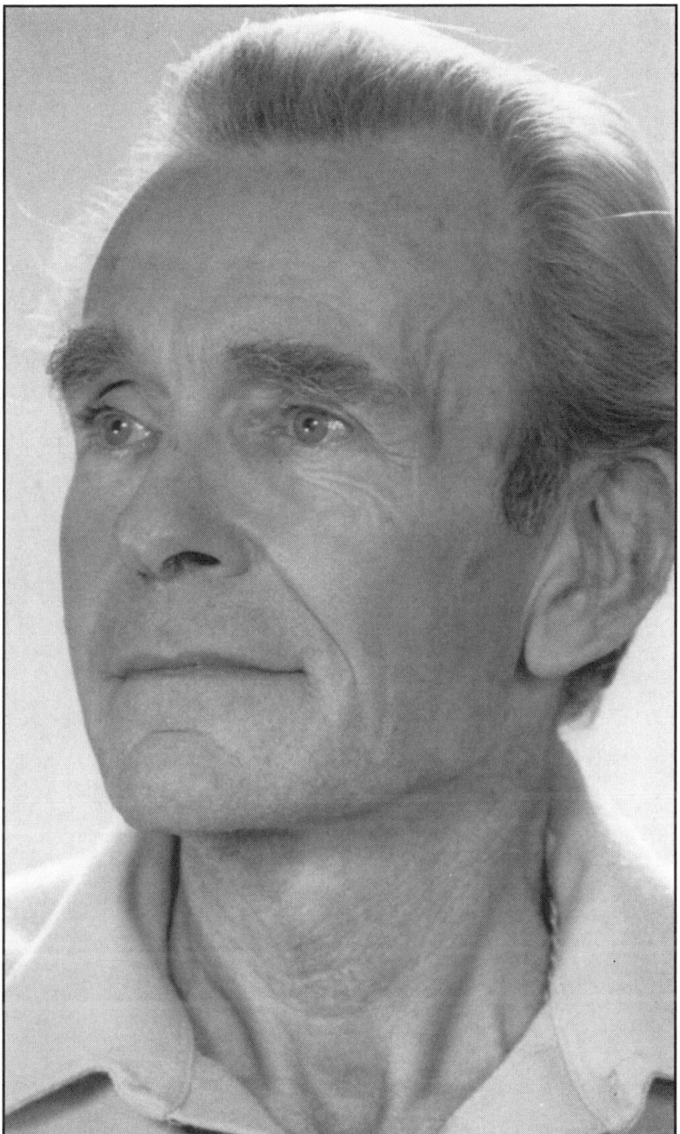

Deep skin rejuvenation: after.

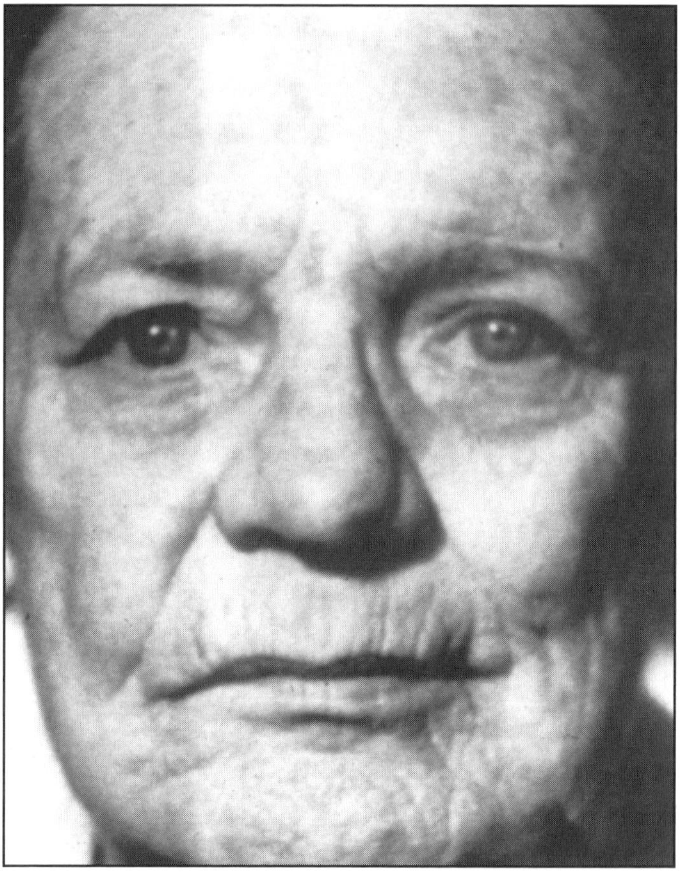

Deep skin rejuvenation: before.

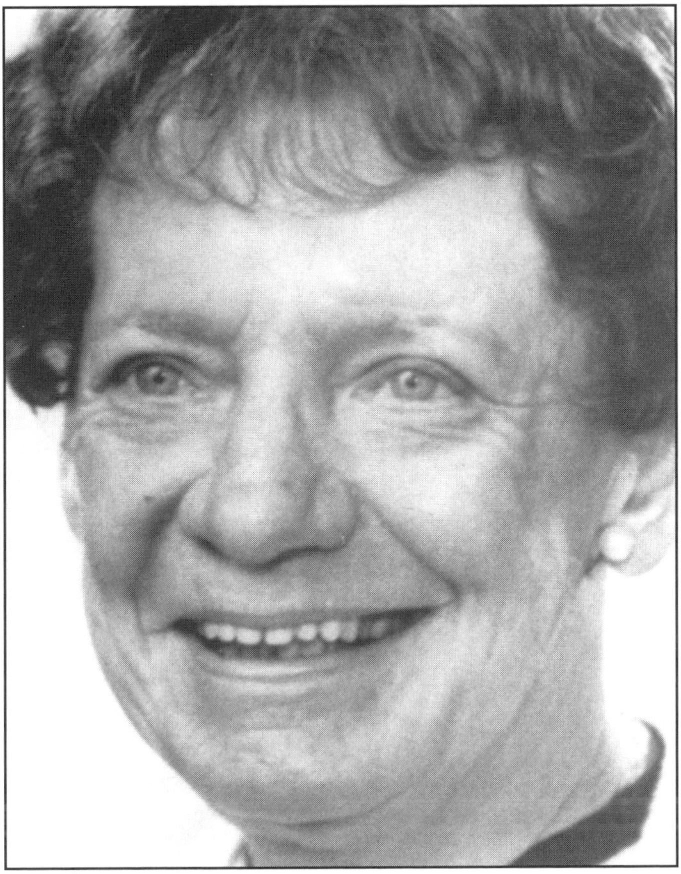

Deep skin rejuvenation: after.

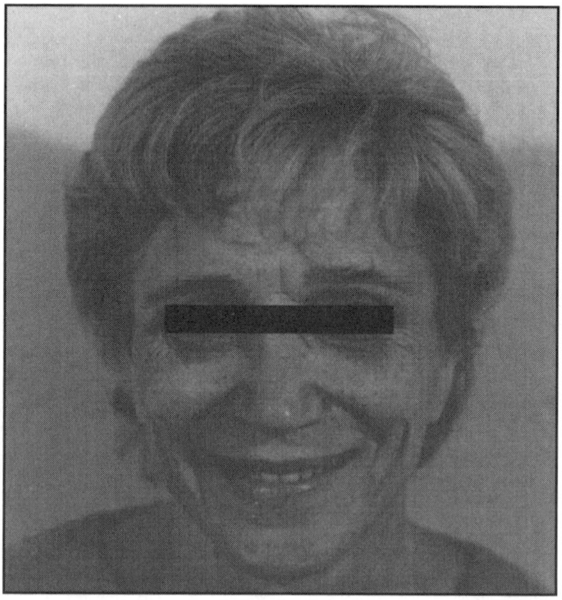

A 64-year-old patient with hyperpigmentation and photoaging

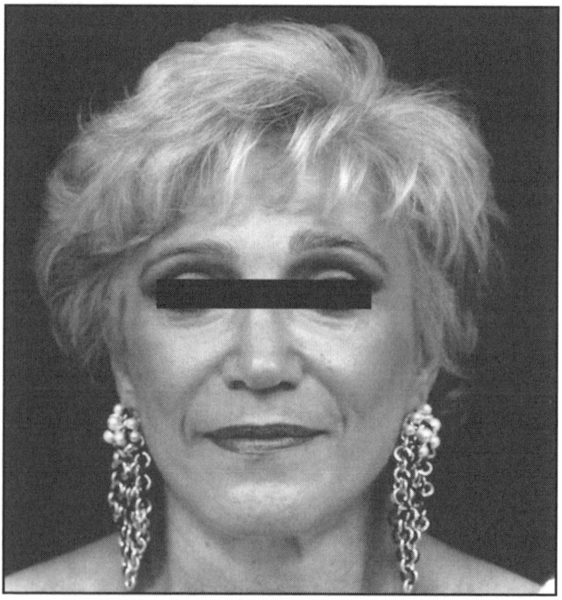

Same patient three months after a deep peel
(She is wearing makeup)

Complications and Side Effects

Chemical peels (chemexfoliation) have proven to be a very effective technique with extremely low incidence of complications, nevertheless, I have to remind you that in any and every medical protocol, complications can and do occur.

Changes in pigmentation, like hyper- or hypopigmentation, are frequent. Hyperpigmentation is especially likely when a patient exposes him- or herself to the sun or takes estrogen during the first six months after treatment.

The most frequent complication is hypopigmentation after a deep peel; many of these cases can be permanent. It is necessary to explain these changes to the patient in order not to have surprises or upset customers.

Infections

In my opinion, infections are so rare because phenol, per se, is an antibacterial agent. Virus infections due to viruses like herpes simplex are far more frequent. That is because 16 to 45 percent of the population has had at least one episode of herpes at some time in their lives.

Milia are small cysts or granules on the surface of the skin that are present one to three months after the peel; normally they auto limit themselves. In some cases, it is necessary to open them and "squeeze them," prolonging redness and swelling.

Redness of the skin is common after a peel; it lasts from six to eight weeks.

Some other changes, such as skin texture, cardiac arrhythmias, and scars around the mouth or the jawline could take place, but your doctor and his or her experience can treat and resolve them.

I think that peels are like "the cake" and other procedures like Botox, fillers, lifters, and even surgery are like the "icing on the cake."

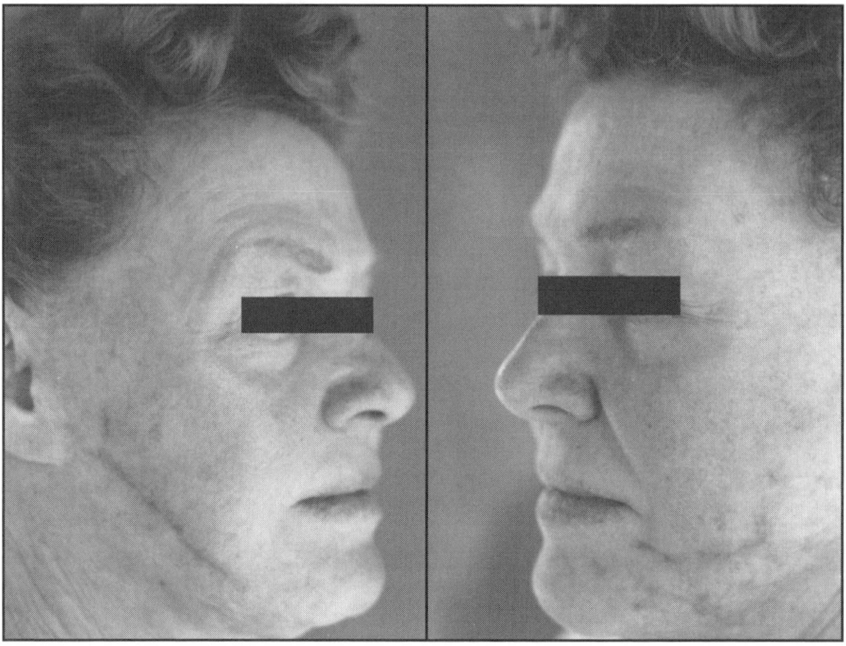

Considerable facial scars due to chemical peel. Hypertrophic scarring on the face after a deep peel—scars that may take months to resolve—are due to poor medical technique.

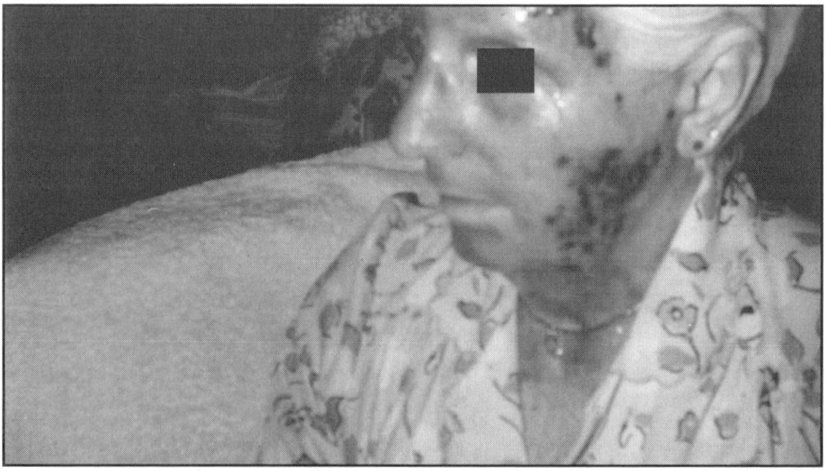

Severe bacterial infection in a 68-year-old patient, 10 days after a deep chemical peel.

Dermabrasion

Dermabrasion is a medical surgical procedure in which a brush, crystals, or "diamond fraises" are applied to the skin in order to remove the skin at different depths. This treatment was in vogue by dermatologists during the 1900s, originally to remove the "tattoos" of thousands of victims from the concentration camps in Europe who arrived in New York after the Second World War. This method of treatment is very specific and unique to dermatologists; it is very bloody and requires a full operating room. (We prefer not to write too much about it, because this book is about "noninvasive" procedures).

Radiofrequency

Radiofrequency produces an efficient inflammatory reaction in healthy patients. It is mainly used for facial rejuvenation. Compared with laser treatment, the patient's recuperation is faster. Radiofrequency can be utilized to diminish the action of muscles on the face of the patient (an alternative to Botox injections).

Botox

In recent years, the treatment that has gained the most attention is the Botulinum toxin (Botox). When it is injected in small concentrations, it produces a temporary paralysis of the injected muscles. This is done by chemical interruption of the union of the nerve with muscles. When this product is injected in the face of the patient, we can temporarily eliminate or minimize dynamic wrinkles (character lines).

I am sure that when you read these paragraphs, you know what we are talking about; perhaps you have had Botox injections. Nevertheless, let me illustrate once more. Each bottle of Botox contains 100 units in a powder form (that you can hardly see in the bottle). Once we apply injectable water, we "activate" the product. It is necessary to use it during the next four hours, otherwise it loses its potency. Once injected into the patient, the effect lasts up to six months (if you are lucky).

The patient needs to ask the doctor how many units he or she is going to use in your face and how many areas is he or she going to treat. Preferably, the bottle should be opened in front of you, or at least ask your doctor when did he or she activate the bottle.

As a general rule, no less than 33 units should be used when the forehead and crow's-feet are injected. When you go to one of those famous "Botox parties," if five patients are treated with one bottle, each patient receives only 20 units. There is no such a thing as "cheap Botox." Each unit should be at least ten dollars. The injection of 100 units should produce one thousand dollars. The cost of the bottle to the doctors is roughly four hundred dollars. If the doctor charges less than ten dollars per unit, he or she is working for the pharmaceutical manufacturer (Allergan). Botox is very effective as well for patients who perspire a lot from the armpits, the palms or the bottom of the feet. The main inconveniences are that the product is expensive, it lasts up to six months, and the injections are painful. Finally, Botox is extremely effective in treating migraines.

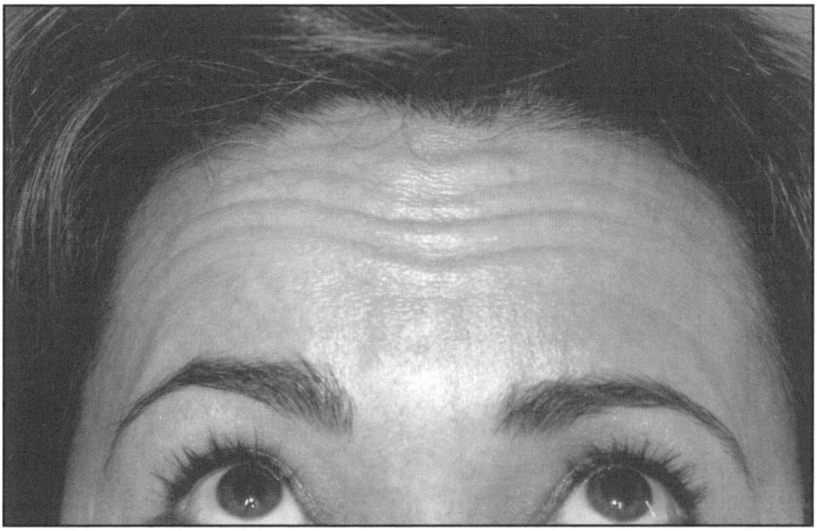

Forehead lines produced by the contraction of the frontal muscle

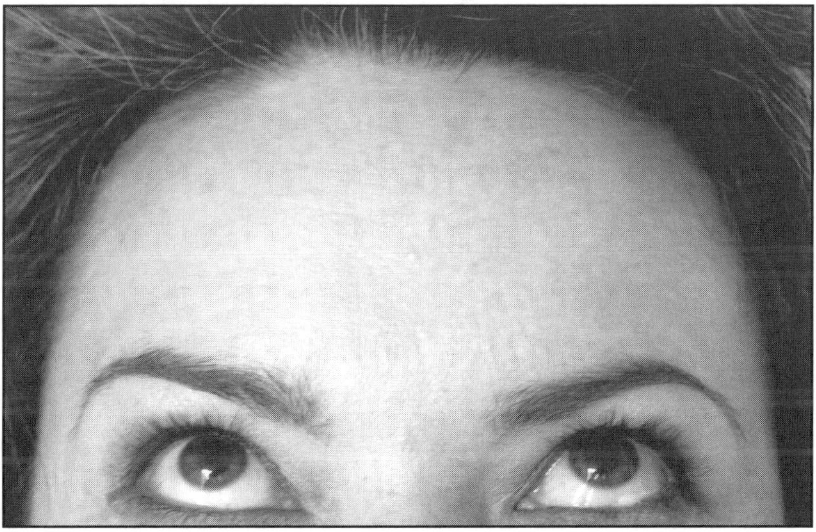

Same patient one week after the application of Botox;
the patient cannot produce the horizontal lines when she tries
to raise her forehead.

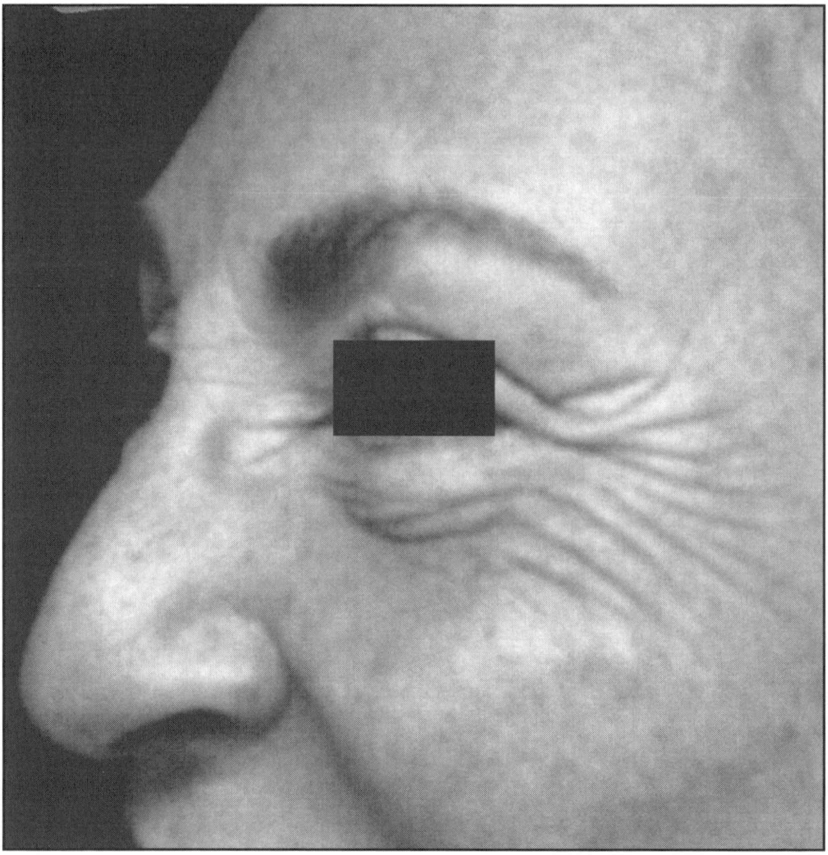

Above. Notice the famous "crow's-feet" when smiling in a patient 67 years of age.

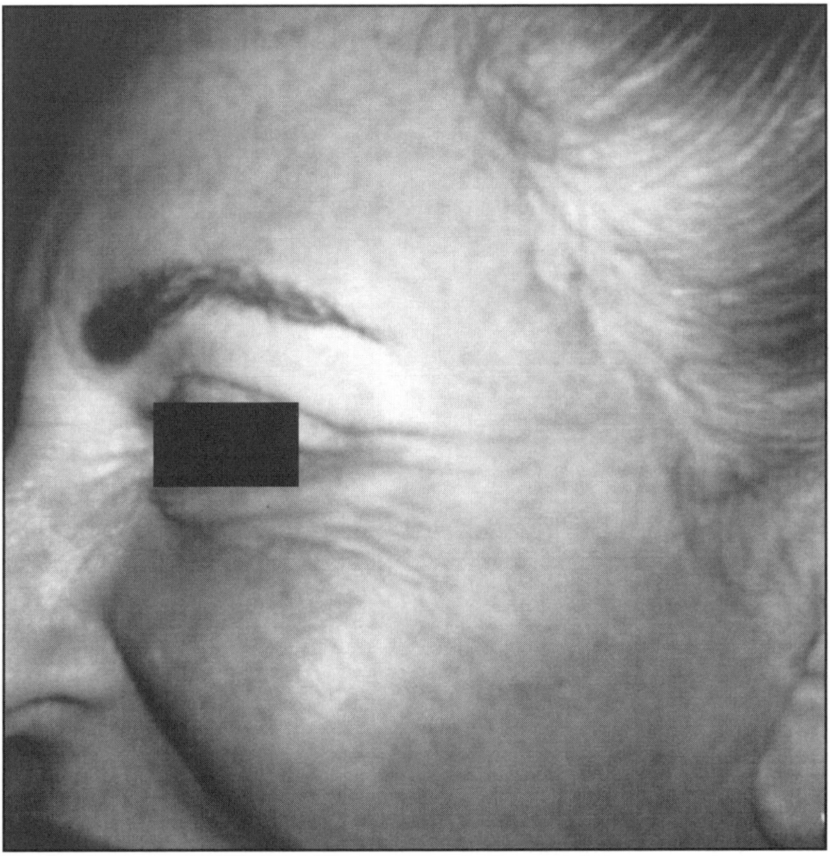

Same patient, two months after the application of 20 units of Botox

Further Reading

Alster, TX, West TB. Resurfacing of atrpophic acne scars with a high energy, pulsed CO2 laser. *Dermatol Surg* 1996:22: 151-155

Alster TS. Comparison of two high-energy, pulsed carbon dioxide lasers in the treatment of periorbital rhytides. J *Dermatol Surg* 1996; 22:541-545.

Alster TS. Improvement of erythematous and hypertrophic scars by the 585-nm flashlamp-pumped pulsed dye laser Ann *Plast Surg* 1993; 22:541-55.

Alt TH. Occulded Baker/Gordon chemical peel; review and update. J *Dermatol Surg Oncol* 1989; 15:980-993.

Asken S. Unoccluded Baker/Gordon phenol peels; review and update. J *Dermatol Surg Oncol* 1989; 15:980-993.

Baker TJ. Chemical face peeling and rhytidectomy. *Plast Reconstr Surg* 1962; 29:199.

Baker, TJ. Discussion on simultaneously deep-plane face lift and trichloroacetic acid peel. *Plast Reconstr Surg* 199; 93:94-95.

Baker TJ, Gordon HL. The ablation of rhytides by chremical means; a preliminary report. J *Fla Med Assoc* 1961;15:998-108.

Baker TN, Gordon HL. Chemical pee with phenol. In Epstein, Epstein E Jr. eds. Skin Surgery, 6th Edition Philadelpia: WB Saundrs, 2987:423-438.

Becker FF, Langford FPJ, Rubin MG, et al. A histological comparison of 50% and 70% glycolic acide peels using solutions with various pHs. *Dermatol Surg* 1996; 22:463-468.

Blitzer A, Brin MF, Keen ME, et al. Botulinum toxin for the treatment of hyperfunctional lines of the face. *Arch Otolaryngol Head Neck Surg* 1997; 123:389-92.

Brandt FS, Bellman B. Cosmetic use of botulinum A exotoxin for aging neck. *Dermatol Surg* 1998; 24:1232-4.

Brody HJ, Hailey CW. Medium depth chemical peeling of the skin: A variation of superficial chemosurgery. J *Dermatol Surg Oncol* 1986; 12:1268

Brody, HJ. Tricholoracetic acid application in cheical peeling. Operative Techniques Plast Reconstr Surg 1995: 2:127-128.

Brody HJ. Variations and comparisons in medium depth chemical peeling. J *Dermatol Surg Oncol* 1989; 2:127-128.

Carruthers A, Carruthers J. The treatment of glabellar furrows with botulinum A exotoxin. J *Dermatol Surg Oncol* 1990; 16:83.

Carruthers A, Carruthers JDA. The use of botulinum toxin to treat glabellar frown lines and other facial wrinkles. Cosmet Dermatl 1994: 7:115.

Coleman WP, Futrell JM. The glycolic acid 1 trichloroacetic acid peel. J *Dermatol Surg Oncol* 1994; 2076-80.

Coleman WP, Yarborough JM, Mandy SH. Dermabrasion for prophylaxis and treatmentof actinic Keratoses. J *Dermatol Surg Oncol* 1996; 22:17-23.

Collins PS. Trichloroacetic acid peels revisited. J *Dematol Surg Onc*ol 1989; 15:933-940.

Colven RM, Pinnell SK. Topical Vitamin C in aging. In: Ledo A (ed.). *Clinics in Dermatology, Skin Aging and Photoaging* 1996; 1:227-234.

Combes FC, Sperber PA, Reisch M. Dermal defects: treatment by a chemical agent. NY Physician Am Med 1960:56-63.

DiNardo JD, Grove GL, Moy LS. Clinical and histological effects of glycolic acid at different concentrations and pH levels. *Dermatol Surg* 1996; 22:421-428.

Ettre CM Griffin TD Murphy GE, et al. The effects of alpha hydroxy acids on photoaged skin: a pilot clinical, histological and ultrastructural study. J *Am Acad Dermatol* 1966; 34:198-195.

Fitzpatrick RE, Goldman MP, Ruiz-Esparza J. Clinical advantages of the CO 2 lsr superpulsed mode. Treatment of veruca vulgaris, seborrheic keratoses, lentigines, and actinic cheilitis. J *Dermatol Surg Oncol* 1994; 20:449-56.

Fitzpatrick RE, Goldman MP, Sauter NM, et al. P:ulsed carbon dioxide laser resurfacing of photoaged facial skin. Arch Dermatol 1996; 132:395-402.

Fitzpatrick RE, Ruiz FJ, Goldman MP. The depth of thermal necrosis using the CO2 laser; a comparison of the superpulsed mode and conventional mode. J *Dermatol Surg Oncol* 1991; 18:340-344

Fitzpatrick RE, Tope WD, Goldman MP, et al. Pulsed carbon dioxide laser, trichloroacetic acid, Baker-Gordon phenol, and dermabasion: a comparative clinical and histologic study of cutaneous resurfacing in a porcine model. *Arch Dermatol* 1996; 17:340-344

Foster JA, Barnhorst D, Paypay E, et al. The use of Botulinum A toxin to ameliorate facial kinetic frown lines. Opthalmology 1996; 103:618-22.

Garcia A, Fulton JE. The combination of glycolic acid and hydroquinone or kojic acid for the treatment of melasma and related conditions. *Dermatol Surg* 1996; 22:443-444.

Garcia A, Fulton JE. Cosmetic denervation of the muscles of facial expression with botulinum toxin. *Dermatol Surg* 1996: 22:39-43.

Garrett SJ, Robinson JK, Roenigk HH Jr. Trichloroacetic acid peel of molluscum contagiosum in immunocompromised patients. J *Dermatol Surg Oncol* 1992; 19:855-858.

Gaughan RN, Otto RA, Renner GJ, et al. The effect of sterile inflammation on skin flap survival. Otolaryngol Head Neck Surg 1986; 95:90-93.

Glogau RG, Matarasso SL. Chemical peels. *Dermatol Clin* 1995; 13:263-276.

Goldman MP, Fitzpatrick RE. Laser treatment of scars. *Dermatol Surg* 1995;21:685-687.

Greenbaum SS, Krull EA, Watnich K. Comparison of CO, laser and electrosurgery in the treatment of rhinophyma. J *Am Acad Dermatol* 1988; 18:36-368.

Griffiths, CEM, Kang S, Ellis CN, et al. Two concentrations of topical tretinoin (retinoic acid) cause similar improvement of photoaging but different degrees of irritation. *Arch Dermatol* 1995; 131:1037-1044.36-368.

Guyuron B, Huddleston SW. Aesthetic indication for botulinum toxin injection *Plast Reconstr Surg* 1994; 93:924-9.

Hayes DK, Berkland ME, Stambaugh KI. Dermal healing after local skin flaps and chemical peel. *Arch Otolaryngol Head Neck Surg* 1990; 116:794-797.

Heckman M, Schaller M, Ceballos-Baumann A, Plewig G. Botulinum beyond wrinkles. *Dermatol Surg* 1997; 23:1221-2.

Hevia O, Nemeth AJ, Taylor JR. Tretinoin accelerates healing after trichloroacetic acid chemical peel. *Arch Dermatol* 1991; 127:678-682.

Hruza GJ, Dover JL. Laser skin resurfacing. *Arch Dermatol* 1996; 12:51-455.

Humphreys TR, Werth V, Dzubow L, et al. Treatment of photodamaged skin with trichloroacetic acid and topical tretinoin. J *Am Acad Dermatol* 1996; 34:638-44.

Hung VC. Topical tretinoin and epithelial wound healing. *Arch Dermatol* 1989; 125:65-69.

Karam PG. 50 resorcinol peel. *Int J Dermatol* 1993; 32:569-574.

Kligman AM, Baker TJ, Gordon HL. Long-term histologic follow up on phenol face peels. Plast Reconstr Surg 1985; 75(5):652-659.

Kligman AM, Grove GL, Hirose, R, et al. Topical tretinoin for photoaged skin. *J Am Acad Dermatol* 186-15:836-859.

Lawrence NL, Cox SE, Brody HJ. A comparison of Jessner's solution and glycolic acid in the treatment of melasma in dark skinned patients: a double blind study. J *Am Acad Dermatol* 1997 (in press).

Leyden JJ, Lavker RM, Grove G, et al. AHAs are more than moisturizers. J *Geriatr Dermatol* 1995; 3:(Suppl A):33A-37A.

Lowe N, Weider J. Botulinumtoxin for hyperkinetic facial lines: a placebo-controlled study. *Cosmetic Derm* 1995; 8:46-9.

Lowe NJ, Maxwell A, Harper H, Botulinum A exotoxin for glabellar folds: a double-blind, placebo-controlled study with an electromyographic injection technique. J *Am Acad Dermatol* 1996; 35:569-72.

Mandy SH. Tretinoin in the preoperative and postoperative management of dermabrasion. J *Am Acad Dermatol* 1986; 15:878-879.

Matarasso SL Glogau RG, Markey AC. Wood's lamp for superficial chemical peels. J *Am Acad Dermatol* 1994; 30:988-992.

Matarasso SL, Glogau RG. Chemical face peels. *Dermatol Clin* 1991; 9:131-150.

Matarasso SL, Glogau RG. The role of chemical peeling in the treatment of photodamaged skin. J *Dermatol Surb Oncol* 1991; 17"622-623.

Matarasso SL. Cutaneous resurfacing. Seminars in Cutaneous Med Surg, 1996; 15:131-214.

Monheit G. The Jessner's 1 TCA peel: A medium depth chemical peel. J *Dermatol Surg Oncol* 1989; 15:945.

Moy LS, Murad II, Roy RL. Glycolic acid peels for the treatment of wrinkles and photoaging. J *Dermatol Surg Oncol* 1993: 19:242-246.

Naumann M, Hofmann U, Bergma I, Hamm H, Toyka KV, Reiners K. Focal Hyperhydrosis. Effective treatment with intrautaneous botulinum toxin. *Arch Dermatol* 1998; 14:301-4.

Nazarro-Poro M. The depigmenting effect of azelaic acid *Arch Dermatol* 1990; 126:1649-1653.

Nelson BR Fader DJ, Gillard M, et al. Pilot histologic and ultrastructural study of the effects of medium-depth chemical facial peels on dermal collagen in patients with actinically damaged skin. J *Am Acad Dermatol* 1994; 32:475-476L.

Newman J, Brandow K, Petmeckey F. Transconjunctival blepharoplasty with simultaneous lower lid ski peel. *Int J Aesth Restor Surg* 1994; 3:43-52.

Olson EA, Katz HI, Levine H, et al. Tretinoin emollient cream: a new therapy for photodamaged skin. J *Am Acad Dermatol* 1992; 25:214-224.

Philips CL, Combes SB, Pinnel SS. Effects of ascorbic acid on proliferation and collagen synthesis in relation to the donor age of human dermal fibroblasts. J *Invest Dermatol* 1994; 103:228:232.

Ridge JM, Siegle RJ, Zuckerman J. Use of alpha-hydroxy acids in the therapy for "photoaged" skin. J *Am Acad Dermatol* 1990; 23:932.

Robinson JK. Actinic cheilitis. *Arch Otolaryngol Head Neck Surg* 1989; 115:848-852.

Rubenstein R, Roenigk HH, Stegman SJ et al. Atypical keloids after dermabassion of patients taking isotretinoin. J *Am Acad Dermatol* 1986; 15:280-285.

Rubin MG. Chemical peeling as an adjuvant therapy for facial neurotic excoriations. J *Am Acad Dertmatol* 1995; 32:296-297.

Spira M, Gerow FJ, Hardy SB. Complications of chemical face peeling. *Plast Reconstr Surg* 1974; 54:397-403.

Stagnone JJ. Superficial peeling. J *Dermatol Surg Oncol* 1989; 15:924-930.

Stegman SJ. A comparative histologic study of the effects of three peeling agents and dermabrasion on normal and sundamaged skin. *Aesth Plast Surg* 1972; 6:123.

Stegman SJ. A study of dermabrasion and chemical peels in an animal model. J *Dermatol Surg Oncol* 1980; 6:490.

Strimling RB, Rogers GS. Correct Toxin dose, multiple site injections: keys to erasing frown lines. *Dermatol News* 1997; 18:8.

VanScott EJ, Yu RJ. Hyperkeratinization, corneocyte cohesion and alpha hydroxy acids. J *Am Acad Dermatol* 1984; 11:867-879.

Waldorf HA, Kauva AN, Geronemus RG. Skin resurfacing of fine to deep rhytides using a char-free carbon dioxide laser in 47 patients. *Dermatol Surg* 1995; 21:940-944.

Weinstein C. Ultrapulse carbon dioxide laser removal of periocular wrinkles in association with laser blepharoplasty. J *Clin Laser Med Surg* 1994; 12:205-209.

Weiss JS, Ellis CN, Headington JT, et al. Topical tretinoin improves photoaged skin; a double-blind, vehicle -controlled study. *JAMA* 1088; 259:527-532.

Wieder JM, Moy RL. Understanding botulinum toxin: surgical anatomy of the frown, forehead, and periocular region. *Dermatol Surg*. 998; 24:1172-4.

Chapter 3
Injectable Materials (Fillers)

As you already know, humans since early civilization have attempted cosmetic improvements; primitive people used topical vegetable paint in order to "adorn" their faces and bodies. Really, it was not until the second half of the nineteenth century that, thanks to the invention of general anesthesia, those cosmetic procedures became popular and more invasive.

During the twentieth century, the utilization of the patient's own fat became the most popular filler, especially after traumatisms.

Today, doctors continue to take fat from the patient's body, but this is a major procedure, requiring an operating room, and in most cases the effect is only temporary.

Due to the great demand for cosmetic procedures, in 1970, medical factories initiated the production of collagen from bovine animals that was injected into patients. By 1990, Europe and Asia developed other products with longer active duration without the need for skin tests, which the bovine collagen required (because patients could be allergic to the protein).

Filling substances have a major value because they are used as "sculpturing materials," since they can produce significant changes in faces and bodies in only a few minutes. Americans call this procedure "lunch-time treatment."

Now in 2012, there are an enormous number of filling substances (soft tissue fillers), each one with precise indications and side effects.

In my practice of more than thirty-five years, we have used them all, but because of price and permanency we use more "medical liquid pure silica" under the commercial name of Dermagen. We have others like polylactic acid, hyaluronic acid, human fibroblast culture, and polymethyl methacrylate.

In general, the classification is based upon its duration, either temporary or permanent.

Temporary Injectables

If you as a consumer are not sure about the effects on your face, it is better to ask your doctor to inject you with "absorbable materials." The most widely used is polylactic acid (Vicryl) although New-Fill® is also recommended.

Among hyaluronic acids, Juvéderm® (no animal origin) together with Restylane®, Hylaform, AcHyal®, Hyacell, Rofilan®, Reviderm and Macdermol® are the most recommendable.

Collagen is a natural protein of human nature, but bovine (cow) or porcine (pig) origin can be used, too. CosmoDerm®, CosmoPlast®, Fibrel, Fibroquel, Resoplast, Cyderm, Zyplast, Permacol, Fascian, and Autologen are the most popular injectibles.

In absorbable biomaterials, we have fibroblast human culture, which is obtained utilizing fibroblast from the skin of the same patient; commercially the product is called Isolagen.

Nonabsorbable Biomaterials

The main ones are bioactive glasses, methacrylates (PMMA), hydroxyapatites, polyacrylamides, politetrachoroethileno, and silicones.

All of these collections of substances are available under different commercial names, and a variety of laboratories produce them. We call them "biomaterials," and they should have some similar and important characteristics.

They should be biologically compatible, they should not cause cancer or allergies, and they have to be resistant to organic absorption. Our body should not be able to destroy them, no bacteria or virus should grow in them, and they should be easily removable and should not interfere with studies like tomography or magnetic resonance.

Any of these materials should be injected under proper asepsis in consulting rooms. They should be not injected during pregnancy or lactation, and they are prohibited in areas where infections or inflammation exist.

In general, soft tissue fillers have two basic indications.

1) To "fill" pre-existing facial or bodily defects
2) To augment similar areas for aesthetic reasons

Facial Modifications

The principal goals of cosmetic medicine are to restore volume and symmetry.Since the time of Leonardo da Vinci, the face was divided into three parts, from the initiation of the hairline to the tip of the chin, and horizontally he or she divided it in the width of five eyes.

Therefore, the upper, mid, and lower face should be in perfect harmony and should be balanced with the horizontality of the face. Soft tissue fillers play an important roll in this process. They can restore symmetry and volume and diminish facial wrinkles.

If we combine fillers with Botox or peels, the result can be more spectacular and of longer duration.

As an example, soft tissue fillers can be used in the forehead to diminish depressions due to scars or acne and in association with Botox to treat horizontal lines, the deep lines between the eyebrows (constipation lines), and the depression in the temporal areas, which can be greatly improved.

In a similar manner, we can "lift" the external or tail part of the eyebrows, in a temporary or permanent manner.

In the lower eyelids, we can restore volume in the channel where the tears run from the eyes.

In the middle face, we can provide volume in the malar eminence (cheeks) as well as improve lack of volume on the side of the face. "Longish" faces are synonymous with the aging process or long-term diseases. A very characteristic feature of patients with acquired immunodeficiency syndrome (AIDS)—the sinking of the side of the face—is due to fat atrophy.

One of the most successful areas to improve is the nose, especially the dorsum and the tip.

The most popular area is the nasolabial depressions known as smile lines.

The lower face is dominated by the lips, not only in the front view but in the profile. Vertical lines around the mouth, especially when kissing, provide a "Grandma" look, and although nothing is wrong with being a "granny," those lines are not at all romantic or sensual. In many patients, we see these lines even without the lips moving.

Besides, lips represent the most "sensual" part of the face. Almost everybody wants to have fuller and more voluptuous lips (like Angelina Jolie).

When you have a pretty nose and beautiful eyes, we men feel "romanticism" and "love," but sensuality in the face can only be obtained with the lips. Any and all areas of the lips can be modified by augmentation materials (see next photograph).

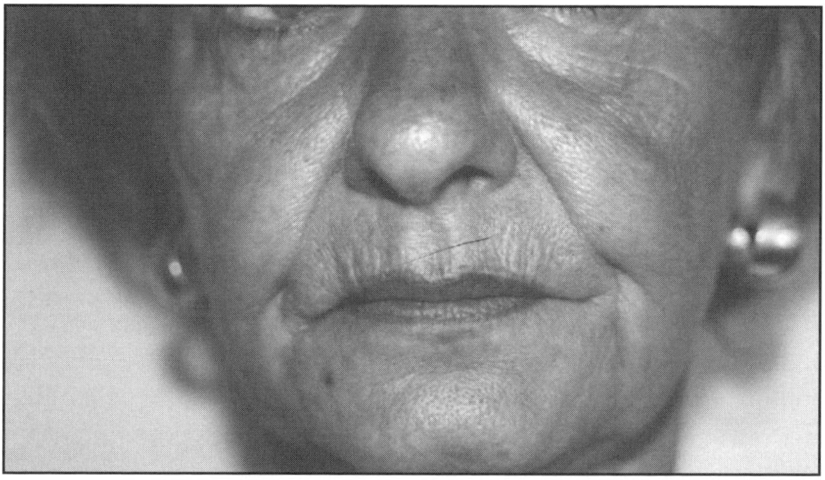

Before correction of vertical lines around lips and nasolabial lines.

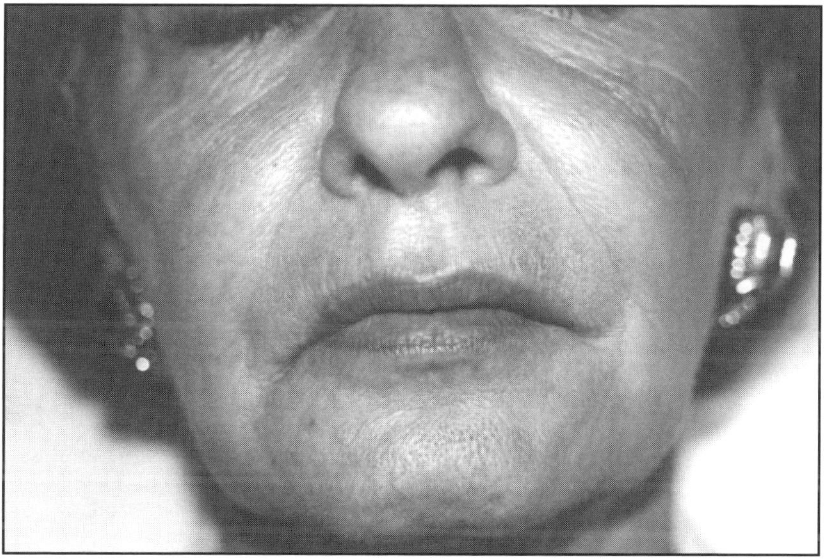

Same patient, after injection of 14 c.c. of permanent filler.

Nice Lips

Do you have a nice pair of lips? Fullness of the lips and strong definition of the philtrum are the main characteristics of nice lips, with 40-60% predomination of the lower lip (pouty).

There is no longer an excuse to have small and insignificant lips. In approximately twenty minutes, we can restore volume and predominance of the lower and upper lip.

"Marionette lines" (corner of the lips to the jawlines) were popularized years ago by the famous dummies like Howdy Doody that moved the lower lip up and down together with the mandible. These depressions can be nicely "filled" in order to minimize signs of aging.

A very strategic area is the chin, which could be short in the front as well as in profile views. This sort of chin accompanied by a prominent "eagle" nose gives what we call "Bird Faces." Nowadays, in a few minutes, without surgery or general anesthesia, we can change both features with extremely pleasant results.

A very important feature is the "jawline." The angle of the jaw can be easily lost with age. A well-pronounced angle provides an "athletic" face just like a superhero. Improved lateral projection can produce well-defined distinction between the skin of the face and the skin of the neck.

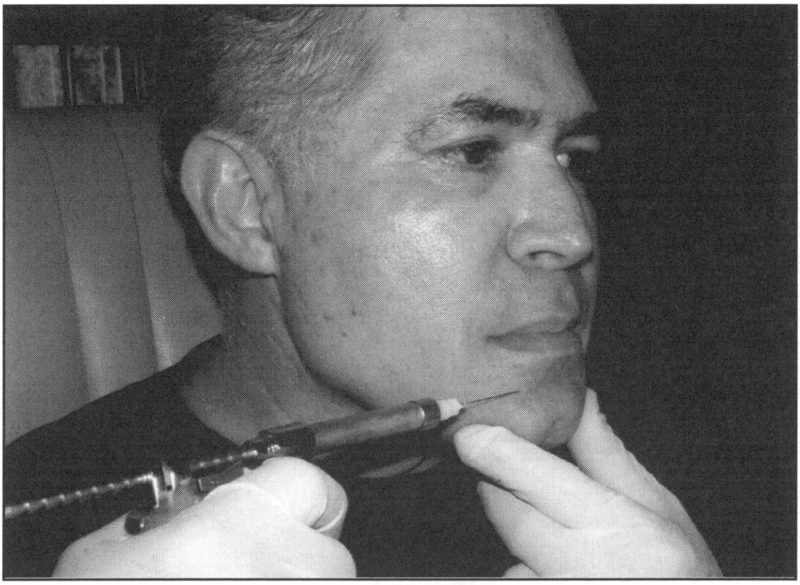

Auto-correction of the chin with injectable filler.
Before: below left. After: below right.

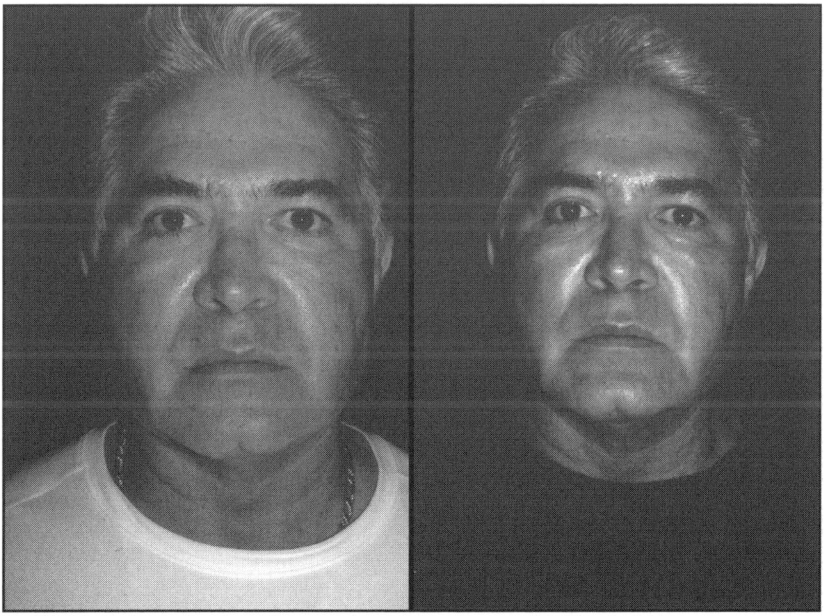

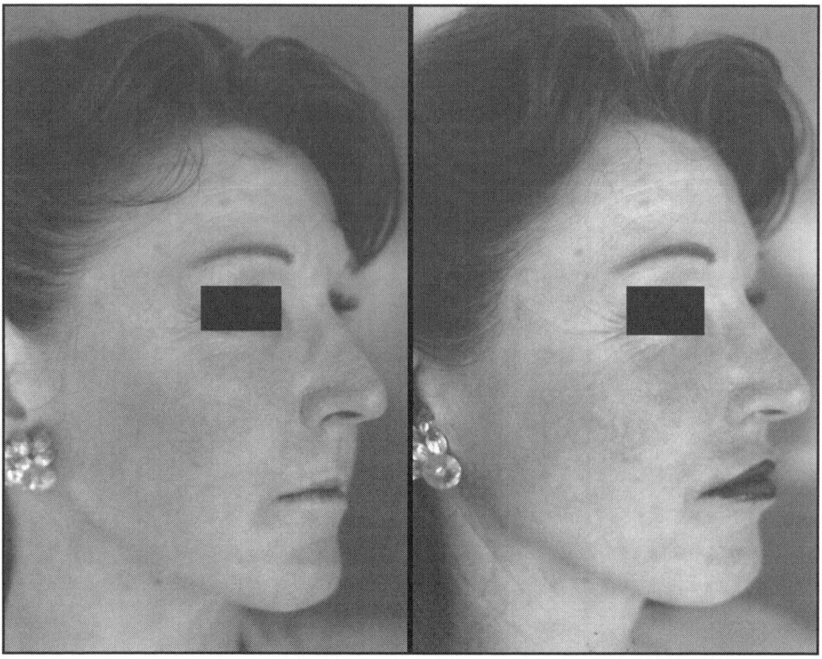

Lip augmentation in a 35-year-old patient
done with 4 c.c. of injectable filler.
Before: left. After: right.

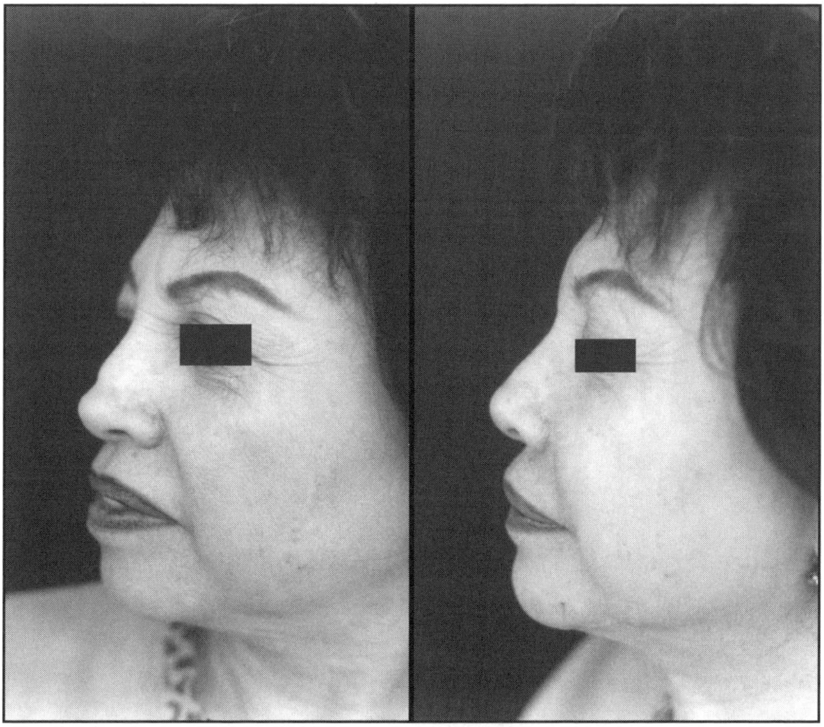

Correction of the cartilege of the nose
done with 2 c.c. of injectable filler
Before: left. After: right.

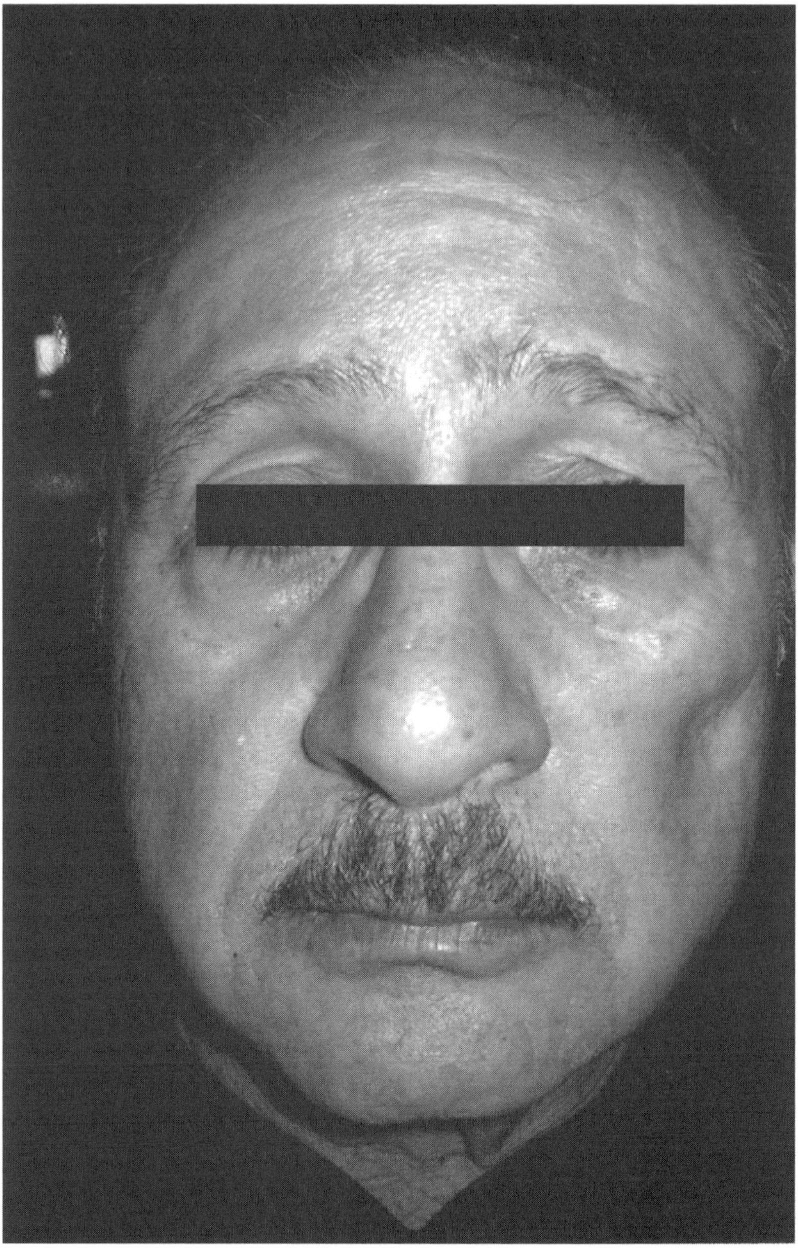

Before: Severe depression on left side of patient's face after an accident.

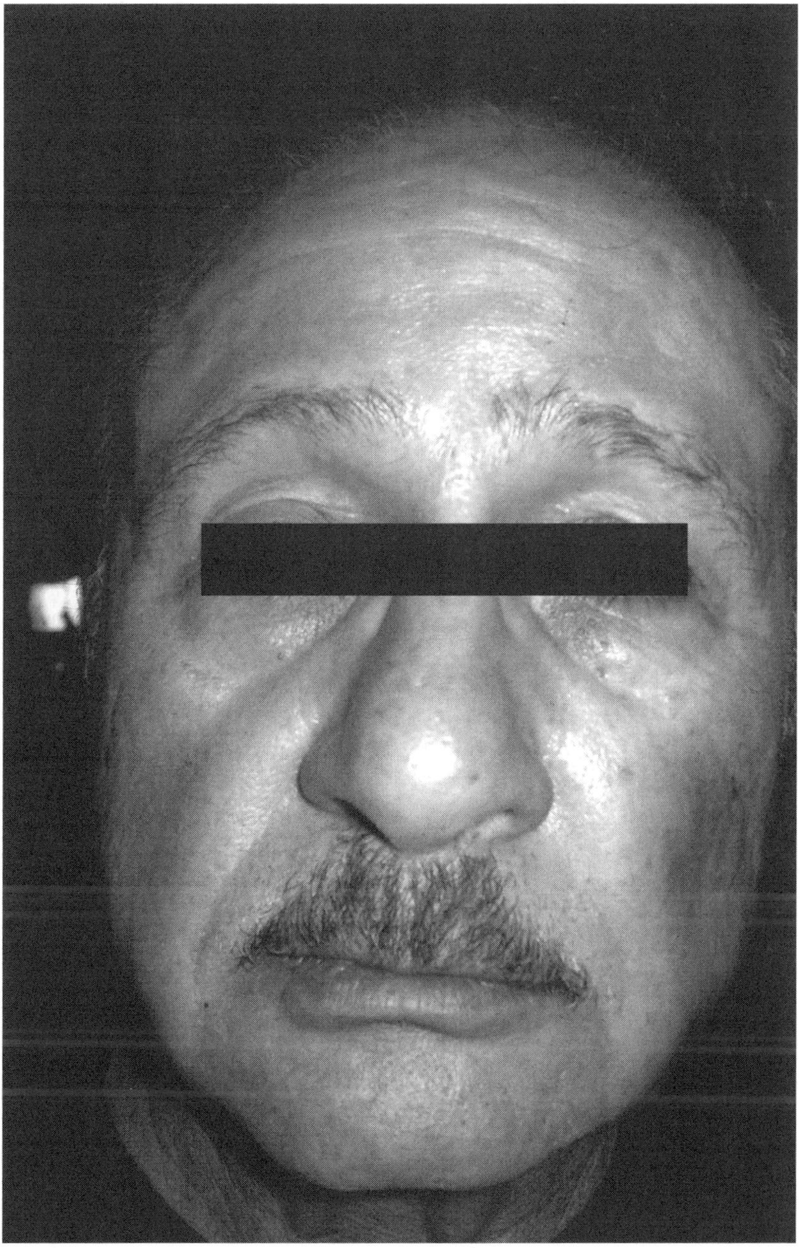

Same patient after the injection of 10 c.c. of permanent filler.

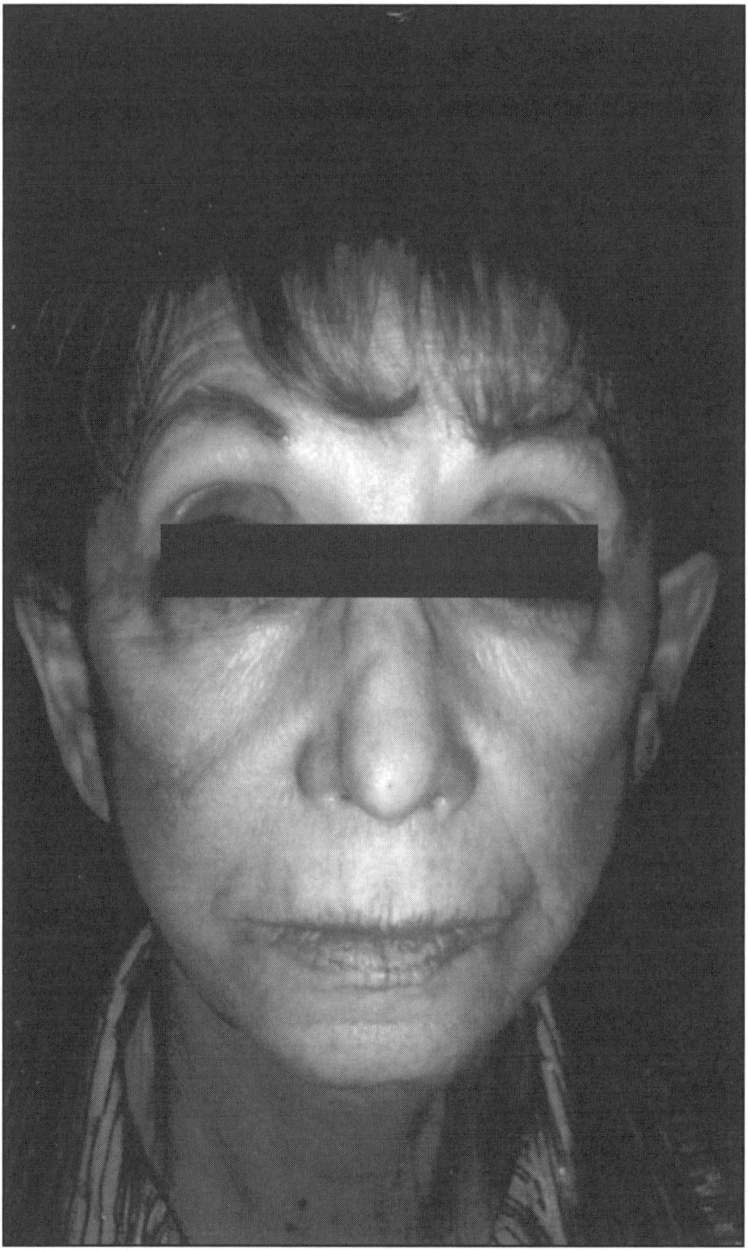

Before correction of the cheeks, jawline, nasolabial lines, marionette lines, and augmentation of the lips.

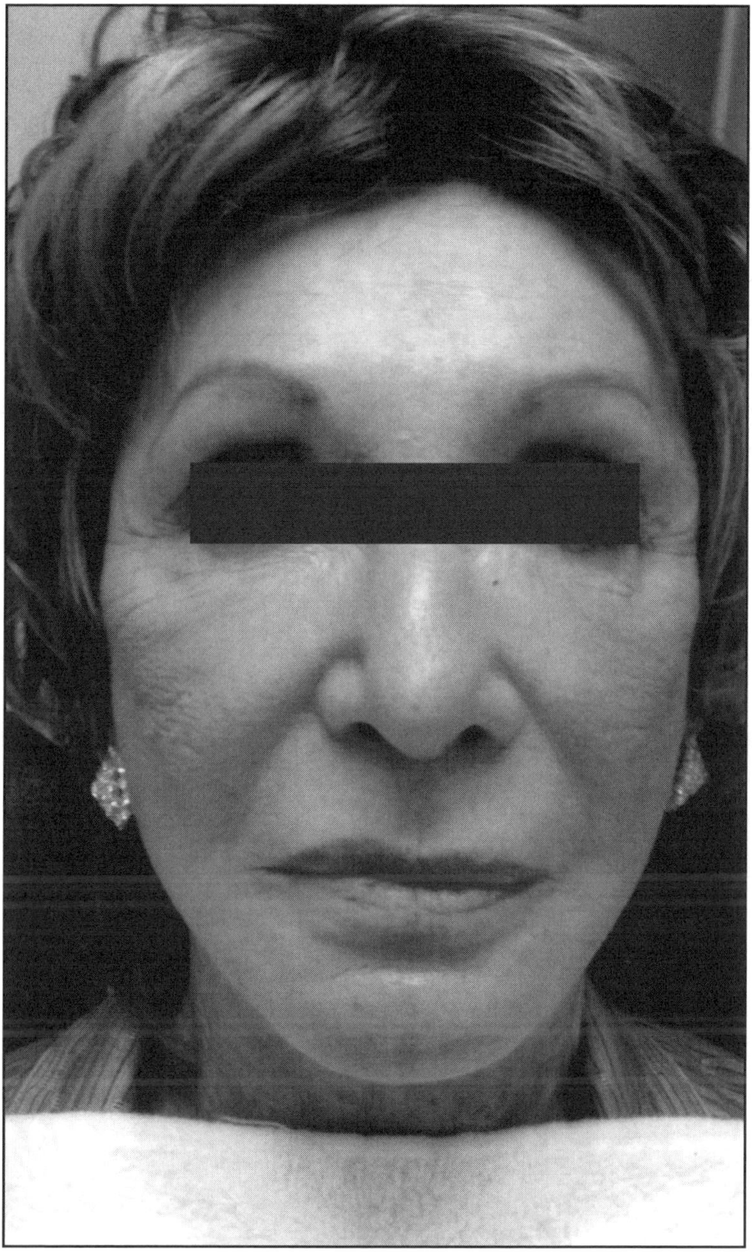

Same patient, transformed with permanent injectable filler.

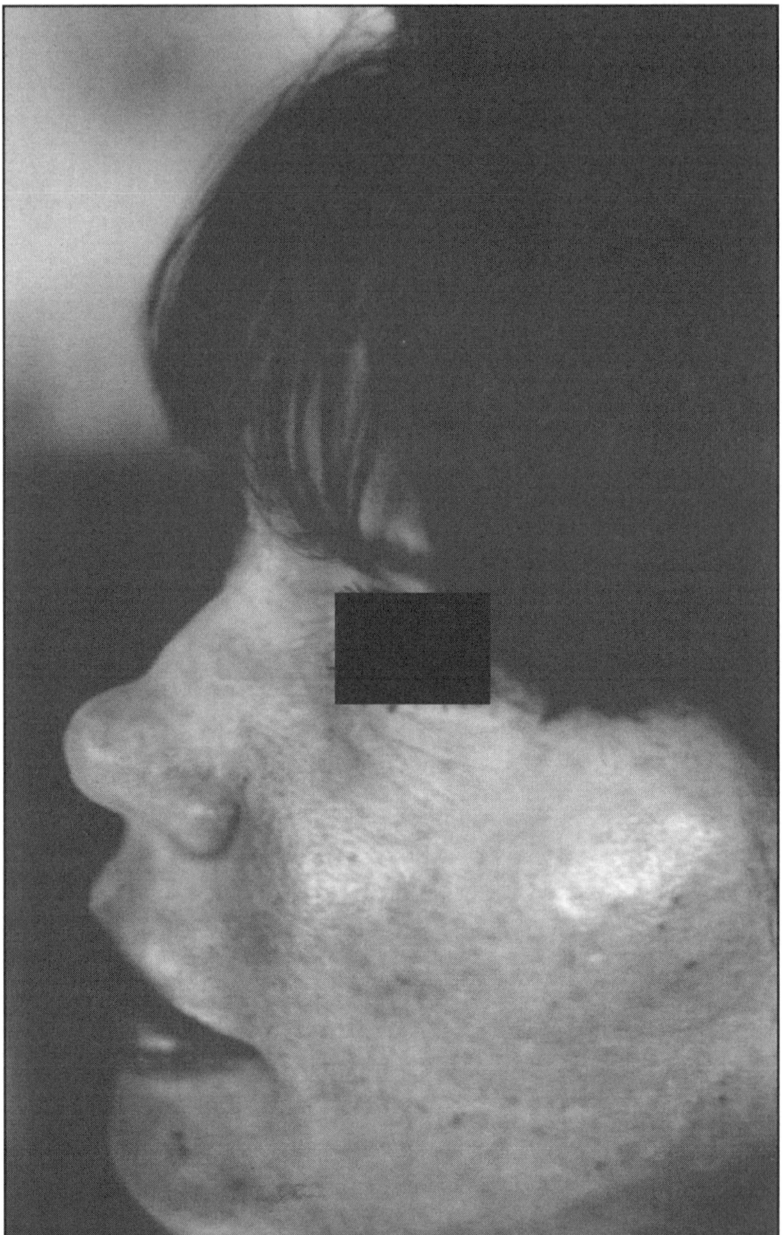

Depression of the nose (saddleback deformity)

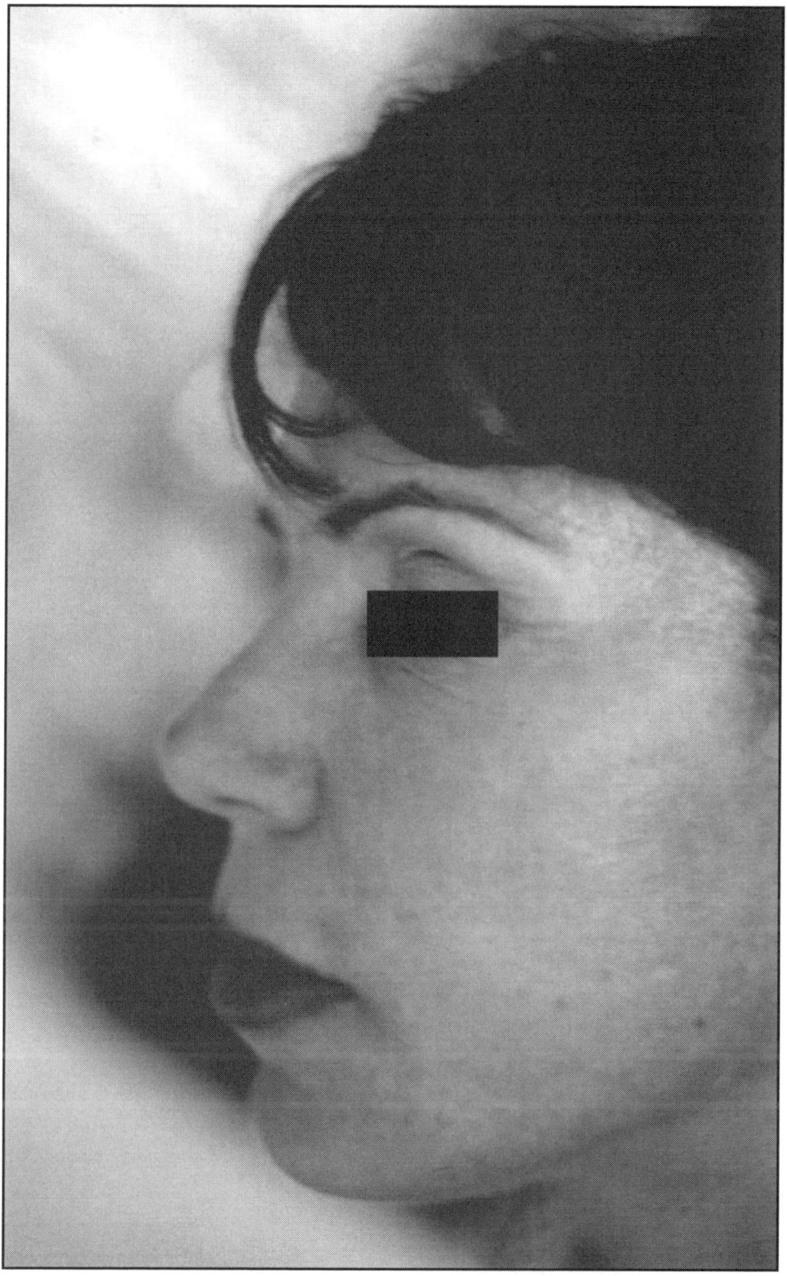

One year after the injection of 4 c.c. of permanent filler.

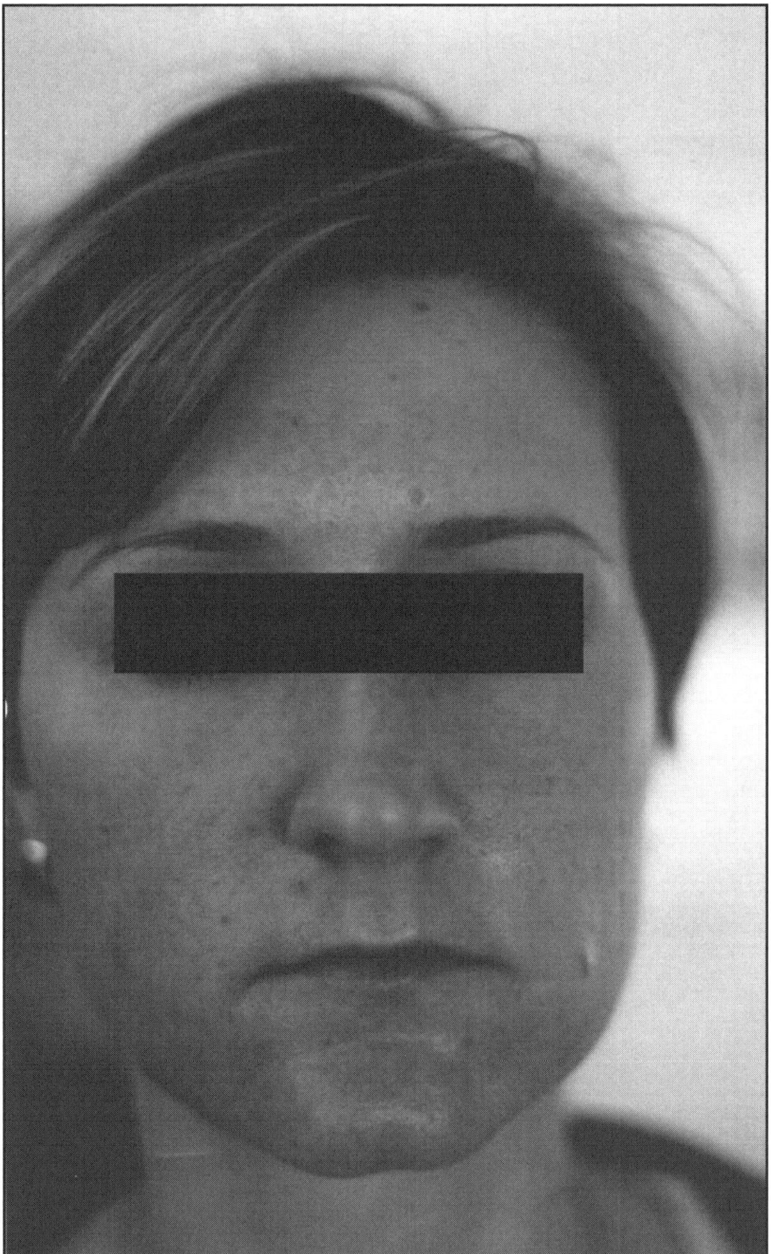

Before: Young woman with thin lips.

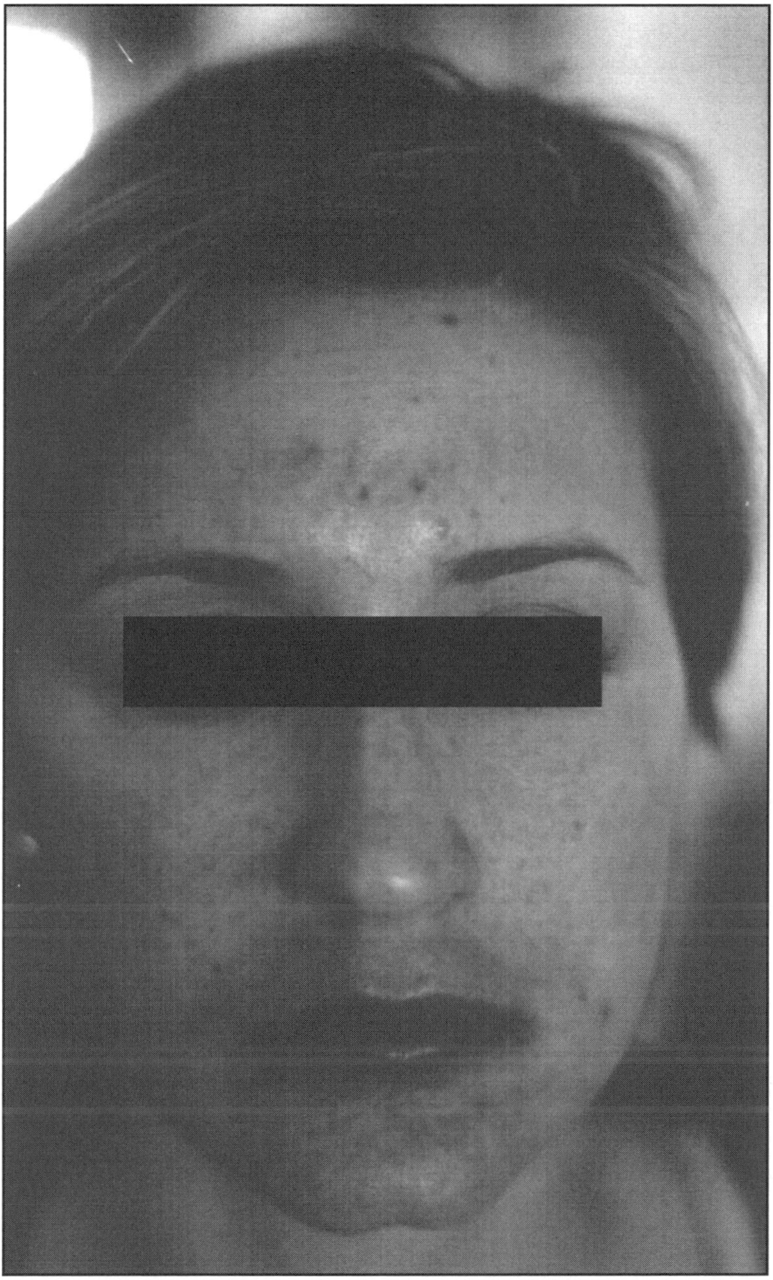

After: Lips enhanced with the injection of 5 c.c. of permanent filler

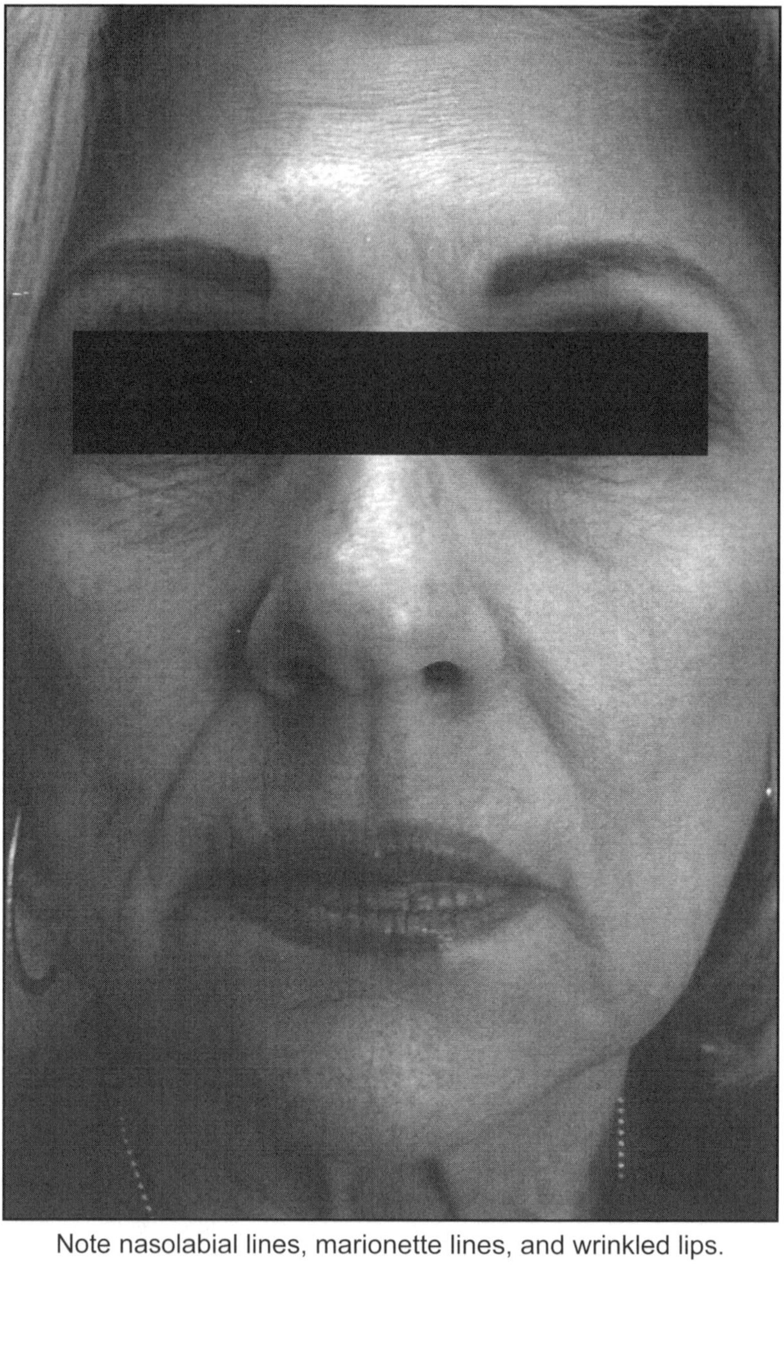

Note nasolabial lines, marionette lines, and wrinkled lips.

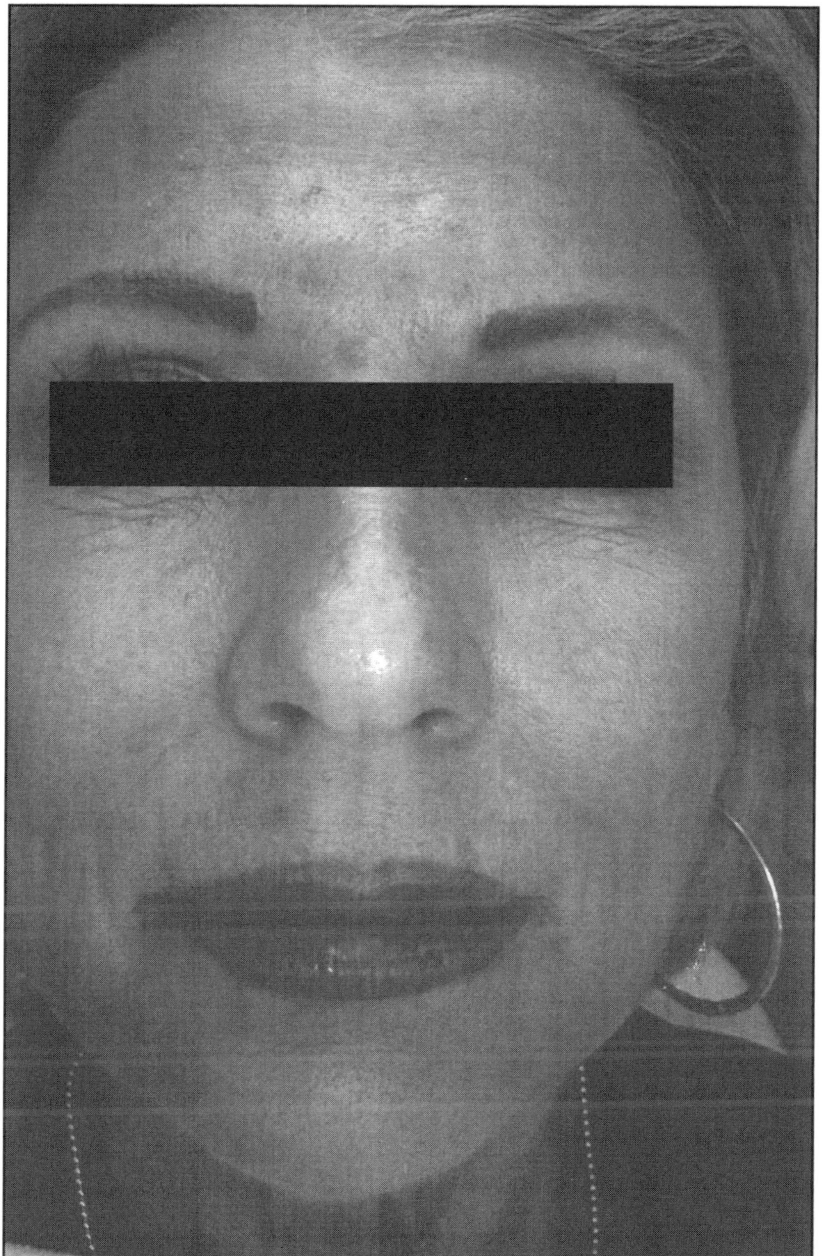

After treatment with 16 c.c. of permanent filler

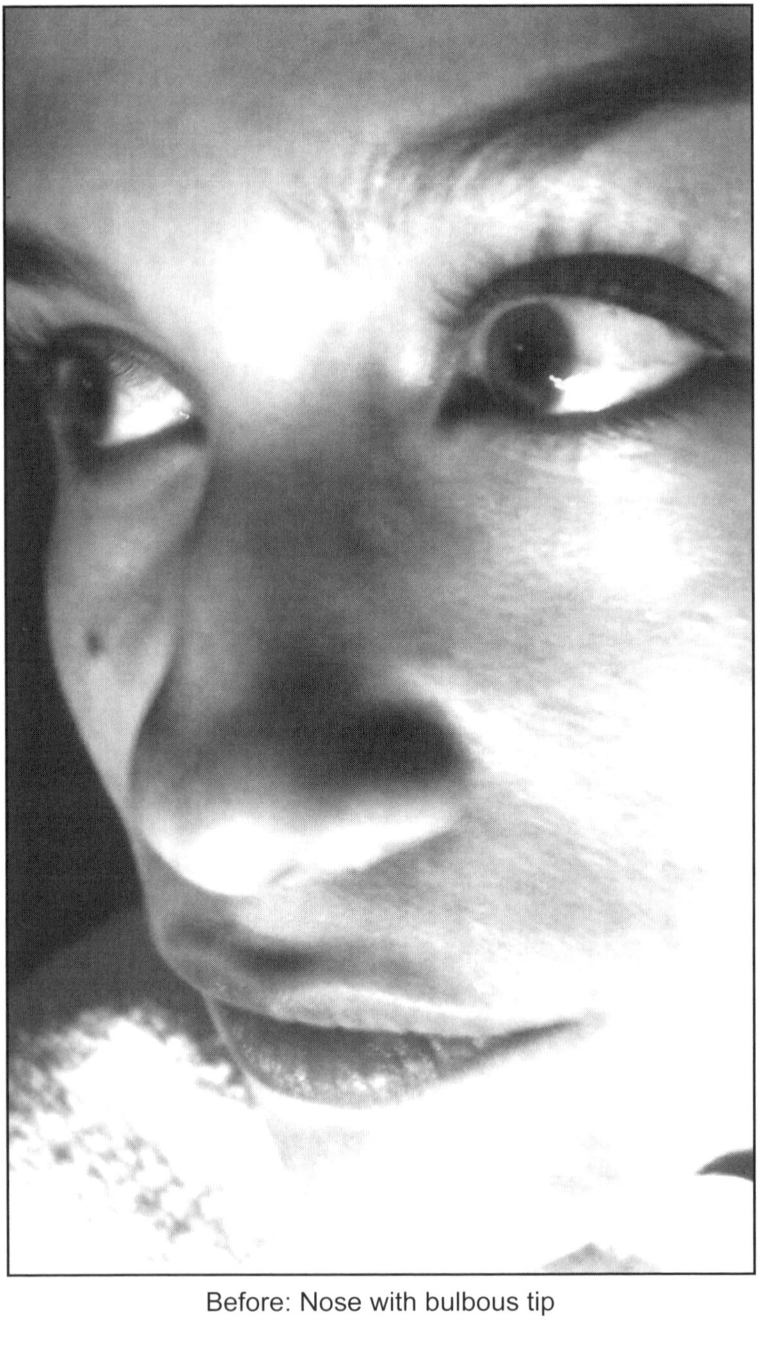

Before: Nose with bulbous tip

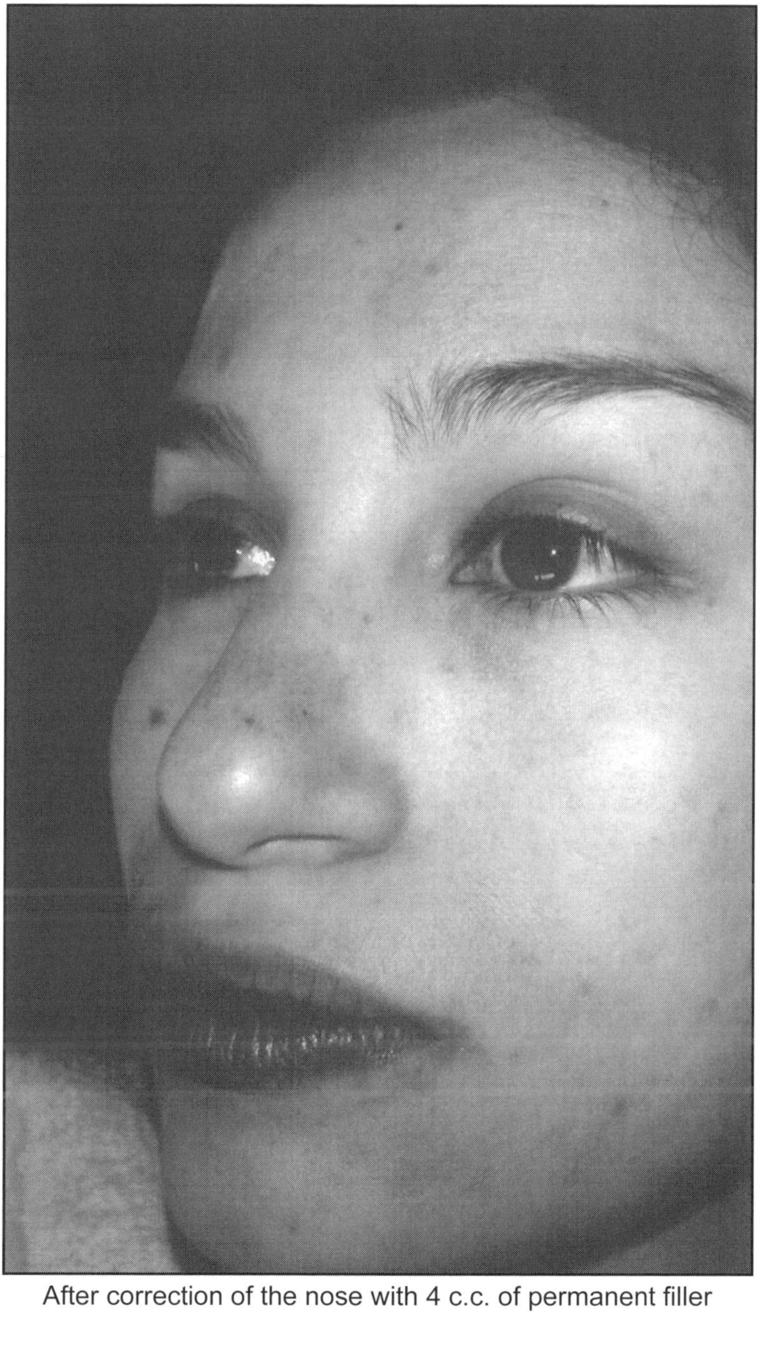

After correction of the nose with 4 c.c. of permanent filler

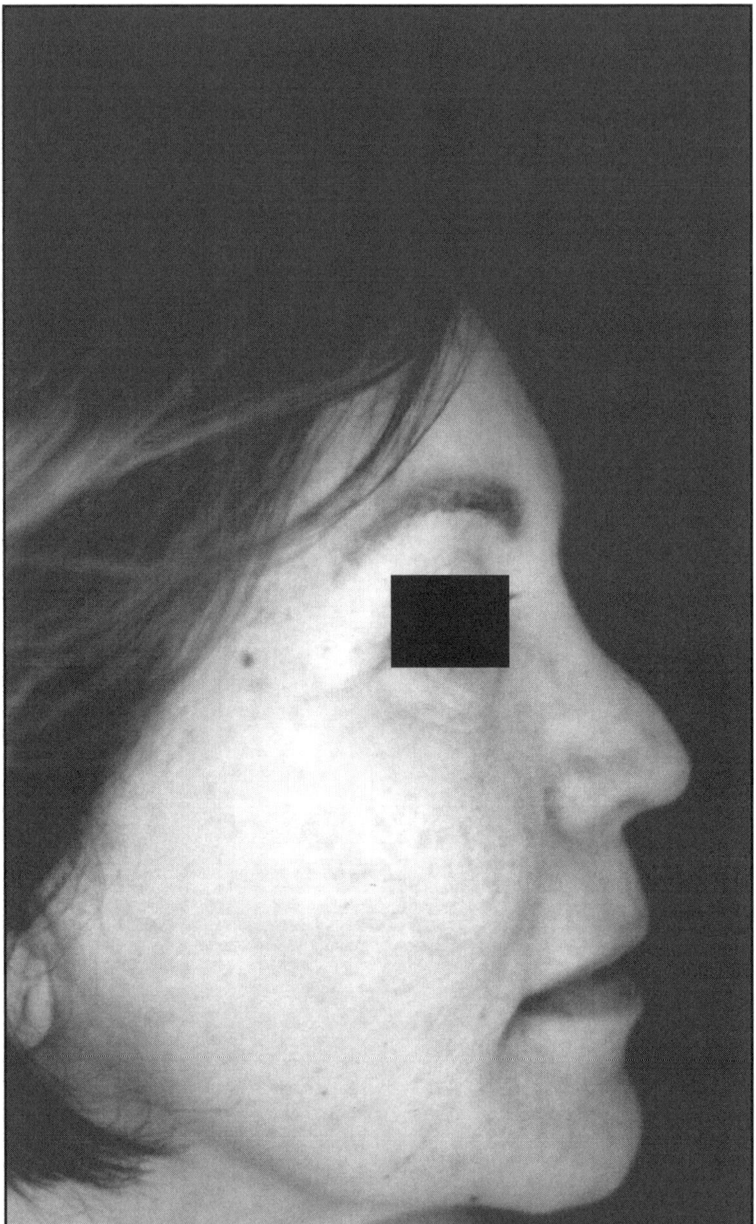

Before

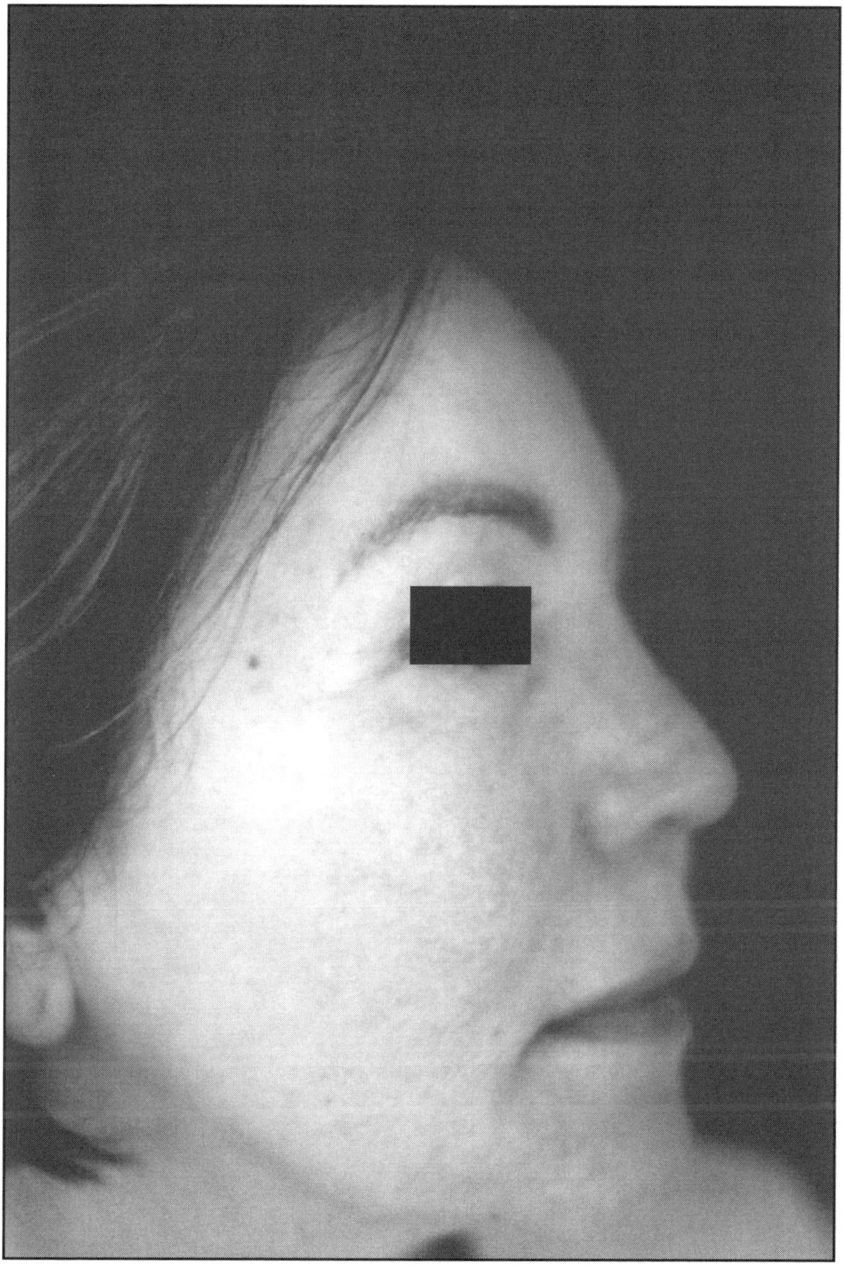

After: Correction of the dorsum of the nose with
2 c.c. of permanent filler

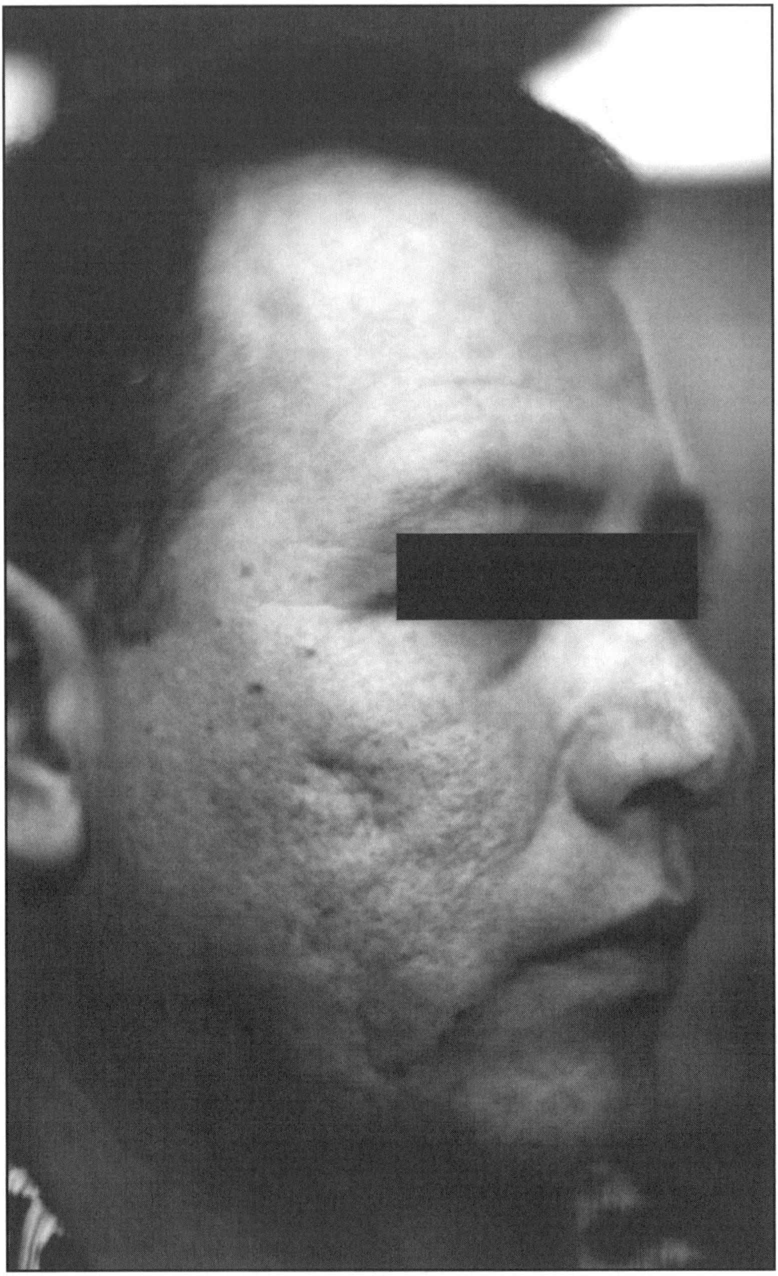

Before correction of acne scars on cheek

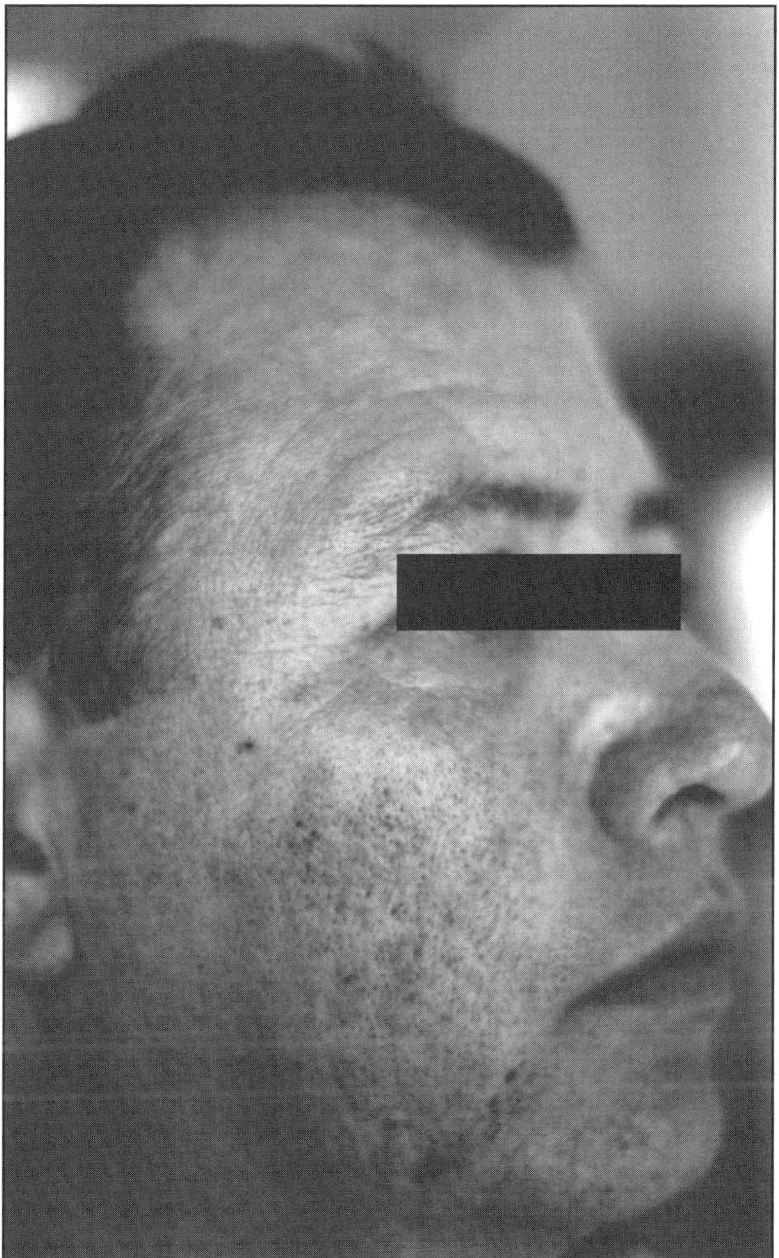

Acne scars after injection of 6 c.c. of permanent filler

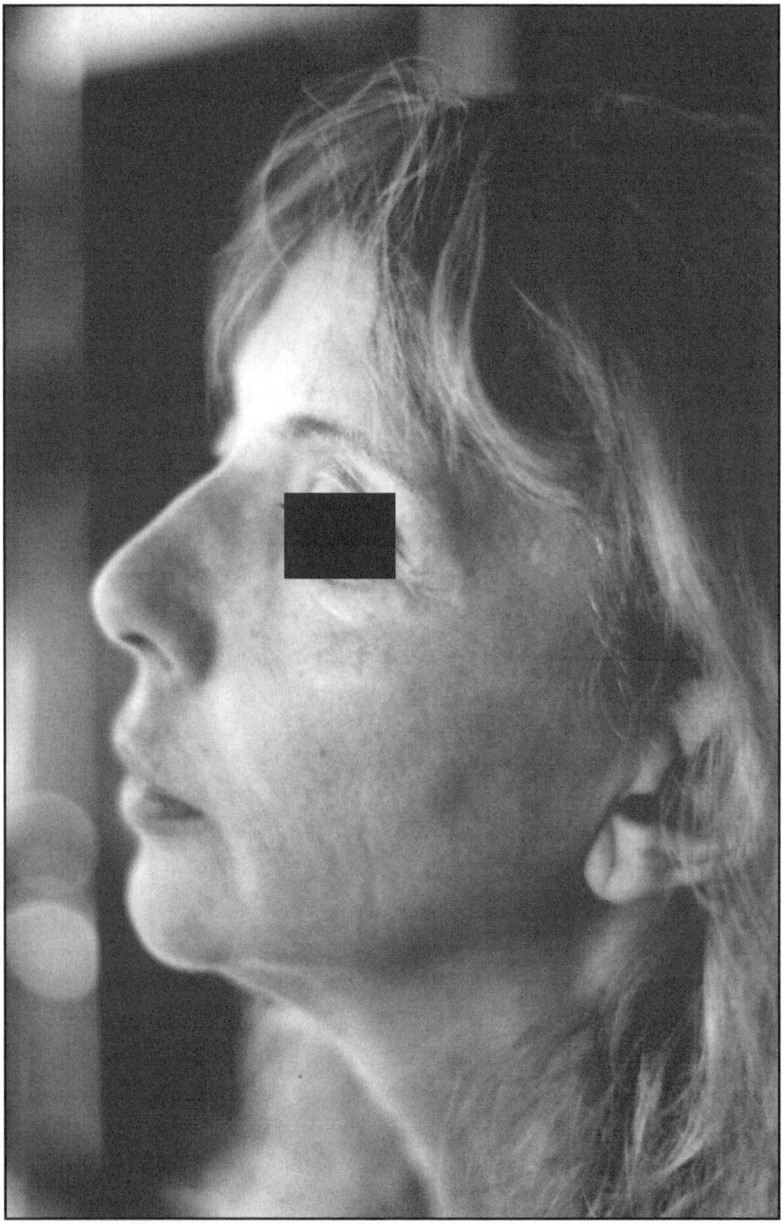

Before lip and chin modification

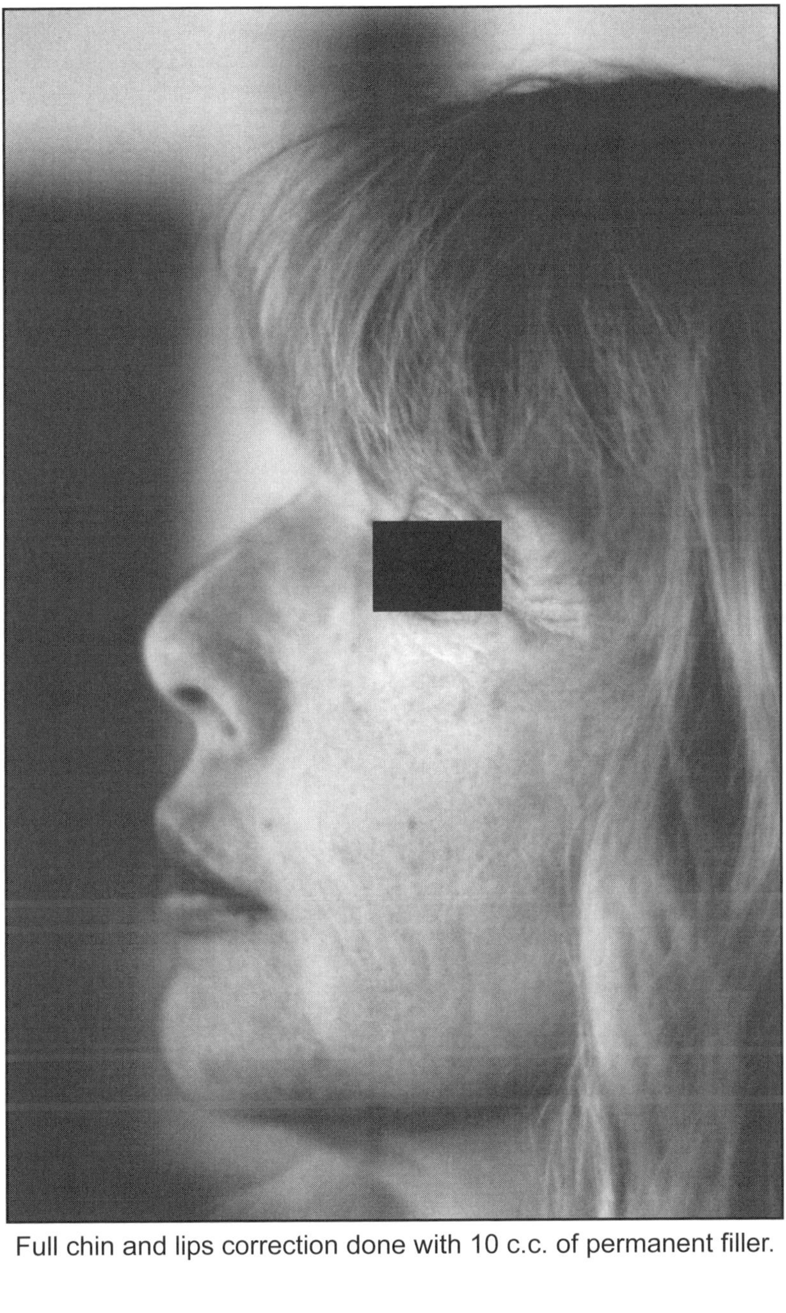

Full chin and lips correction done with 10 c.c. of permanent filler.

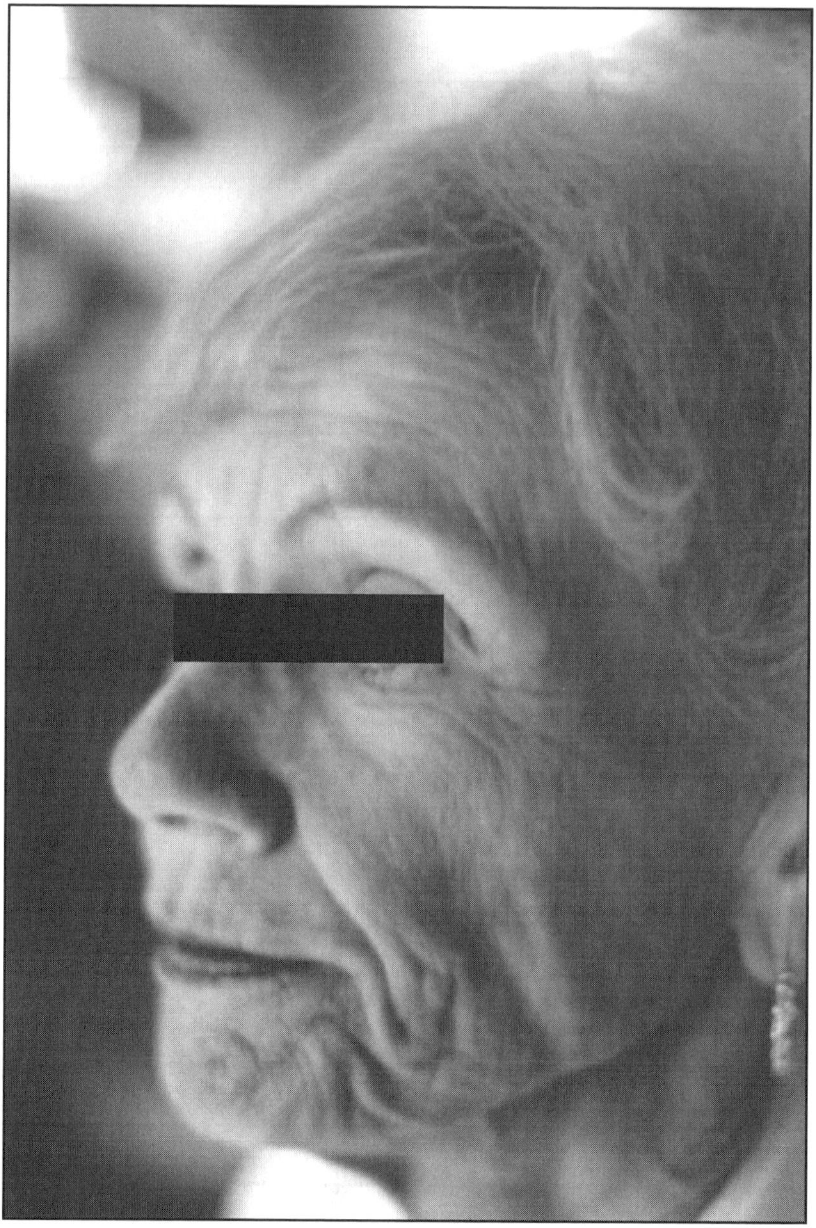

Before: excessive skin folds

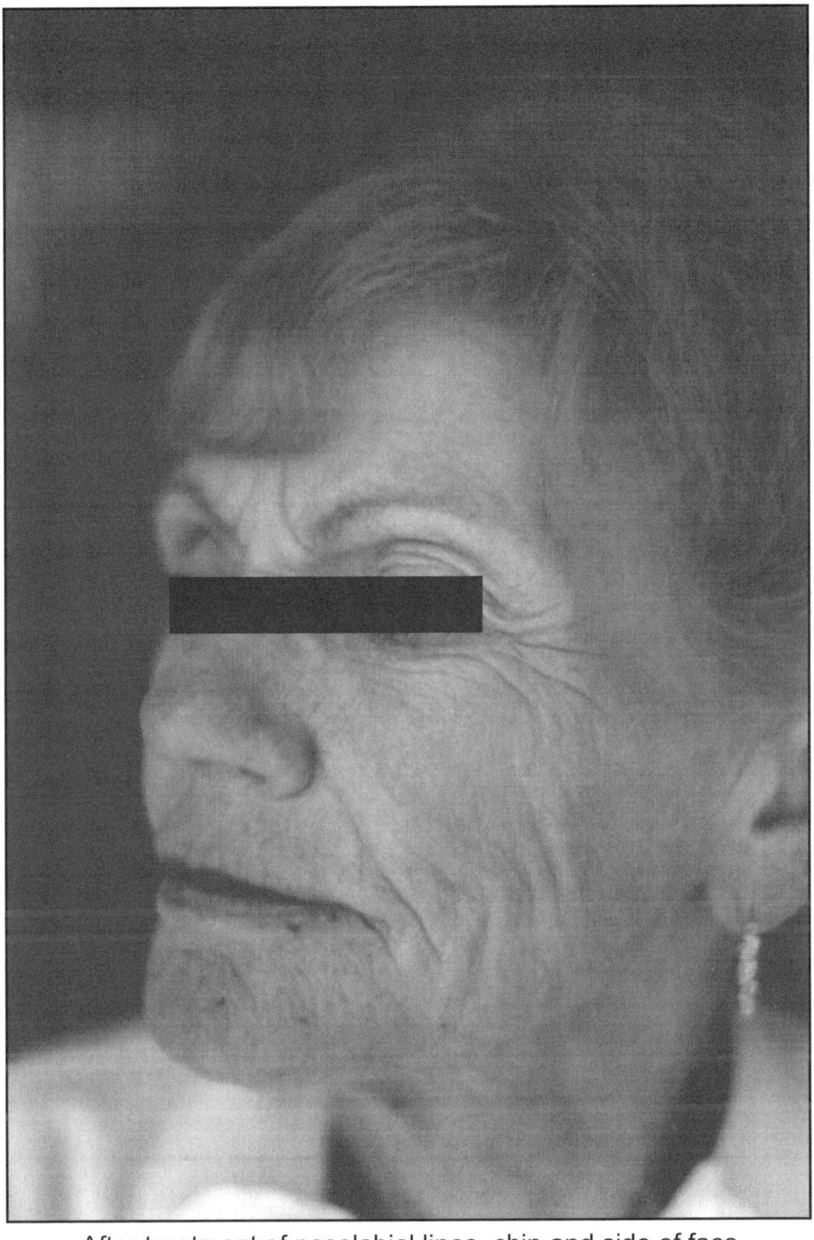

After treatment of nasolabial lines, chin and side of face with 20 c.c. of permanent filler

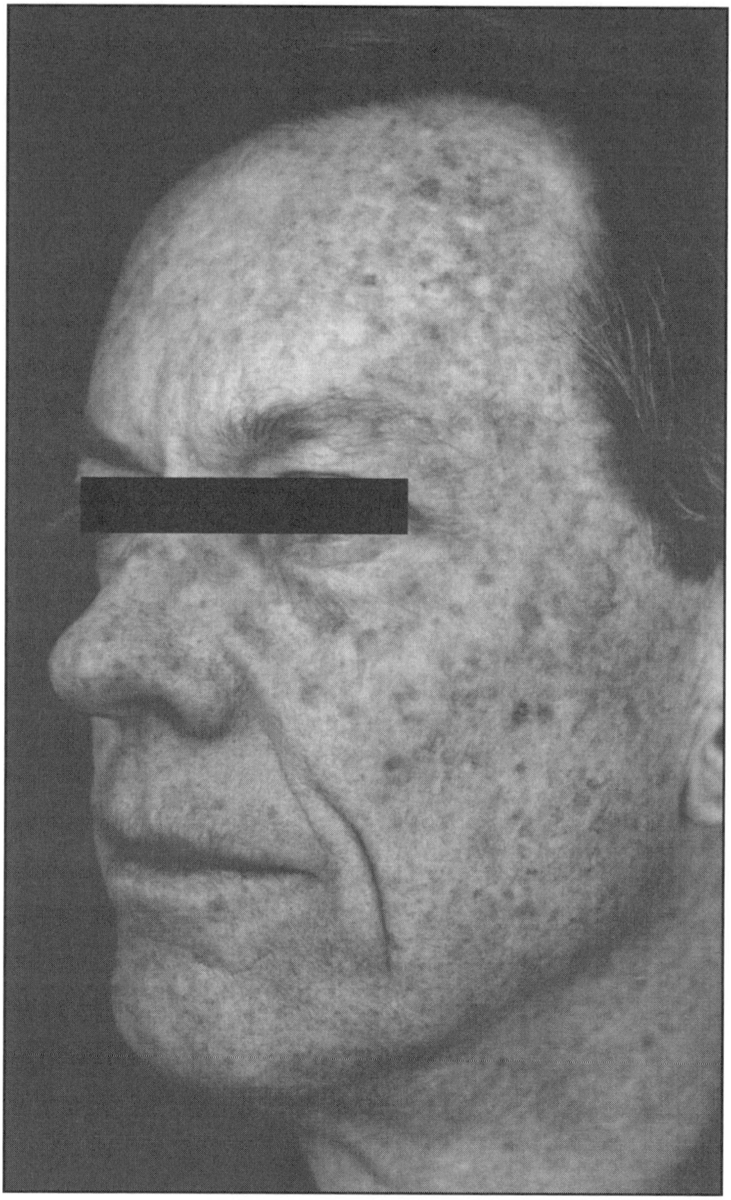

Before: nasolabial folds

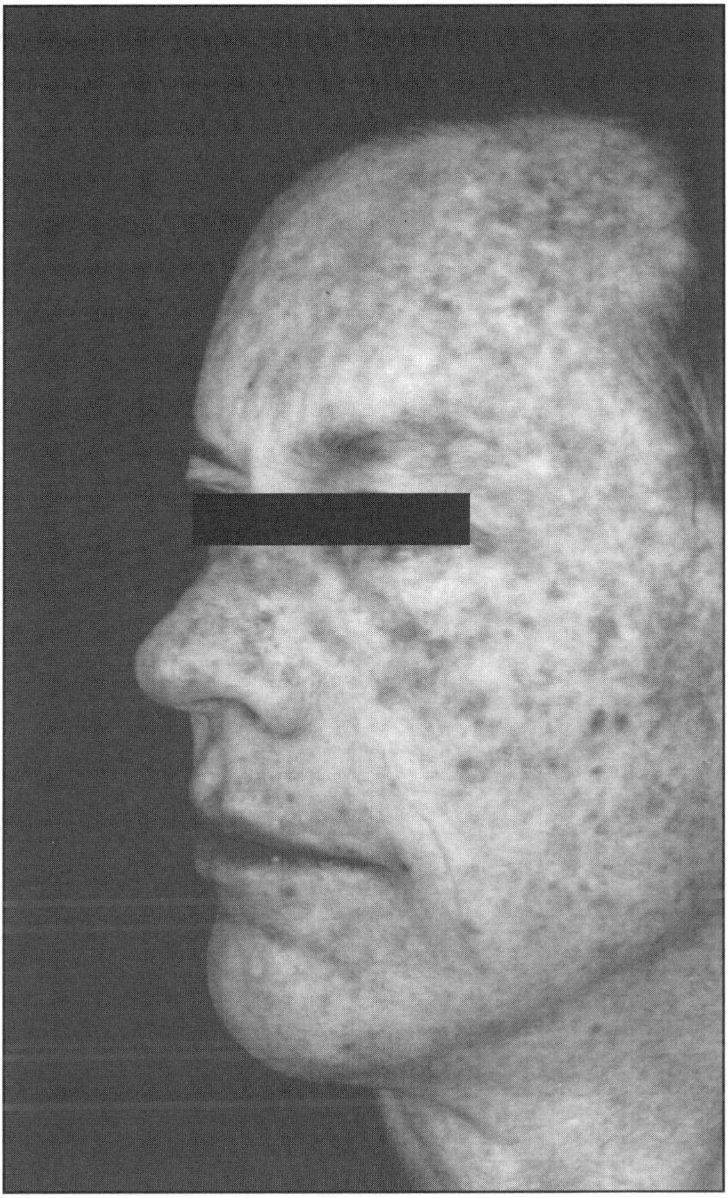

After nasolabial depressions were treated with
15 c.c. of permanent filler

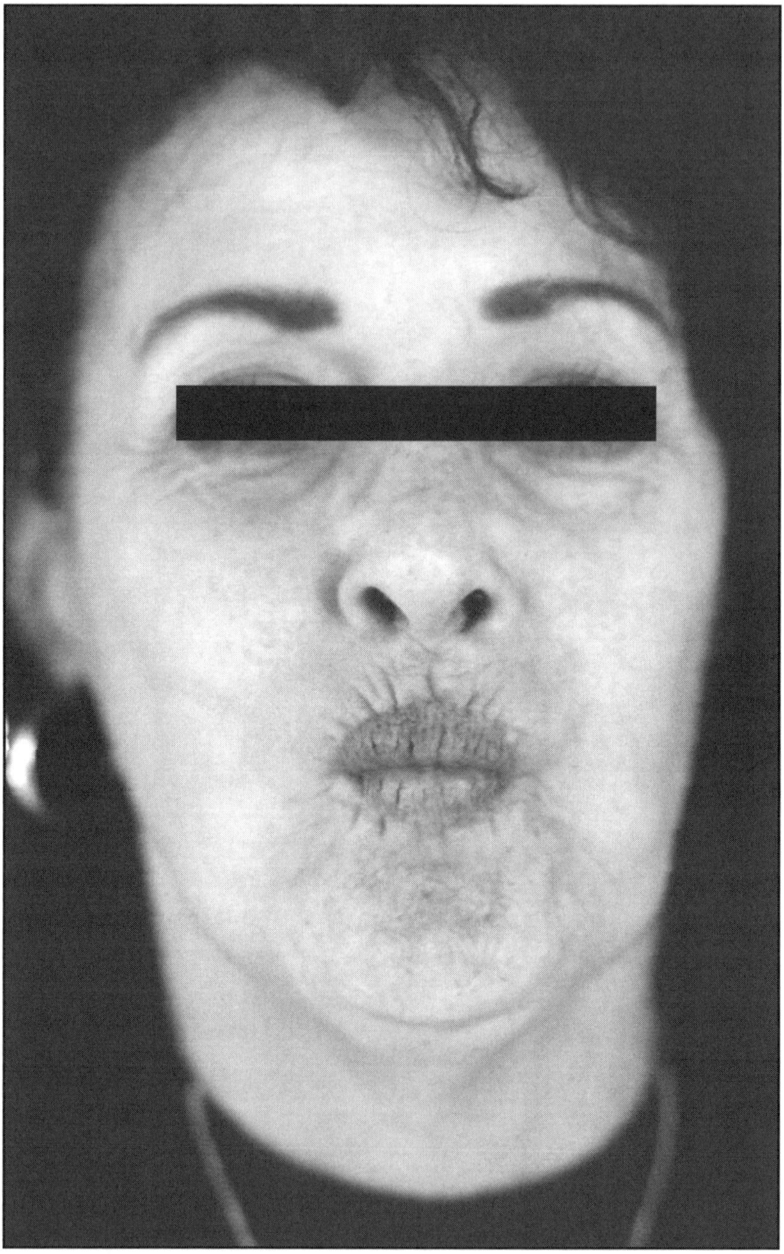

Note vertical lines around lips before treatment

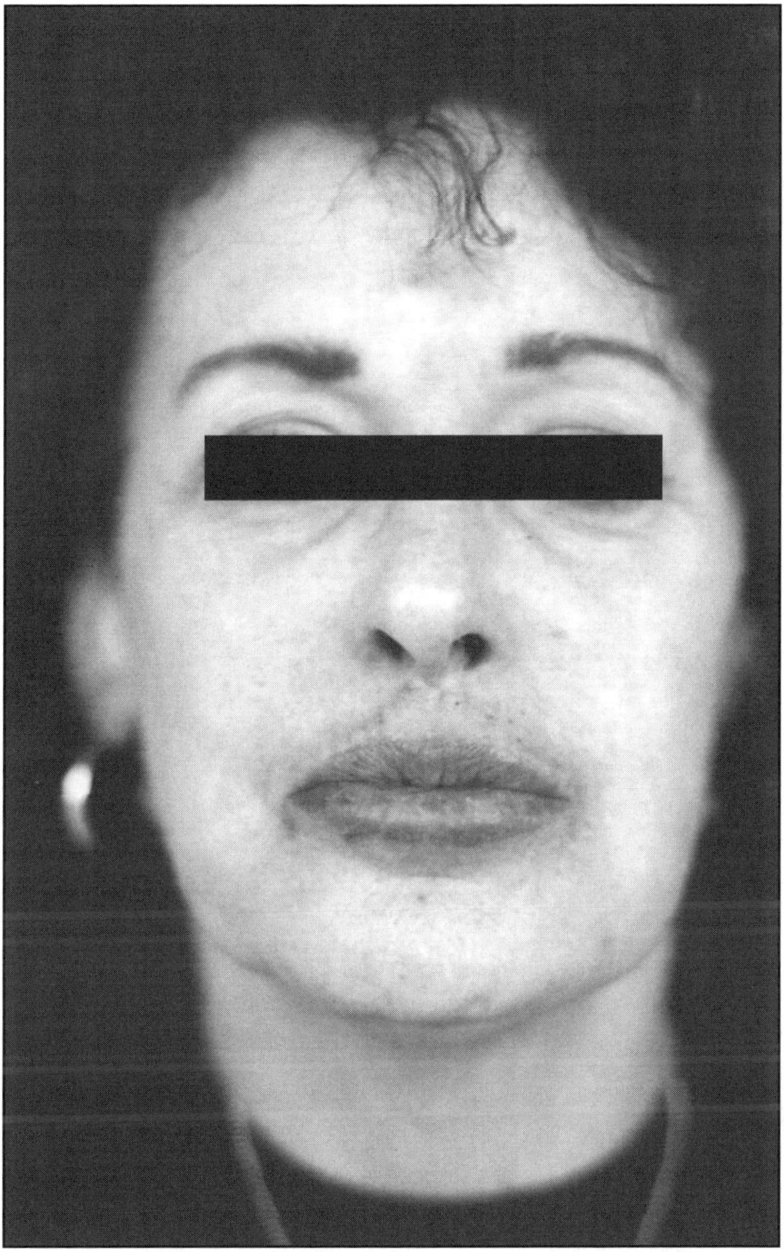

After treatment with injectable permanent filler

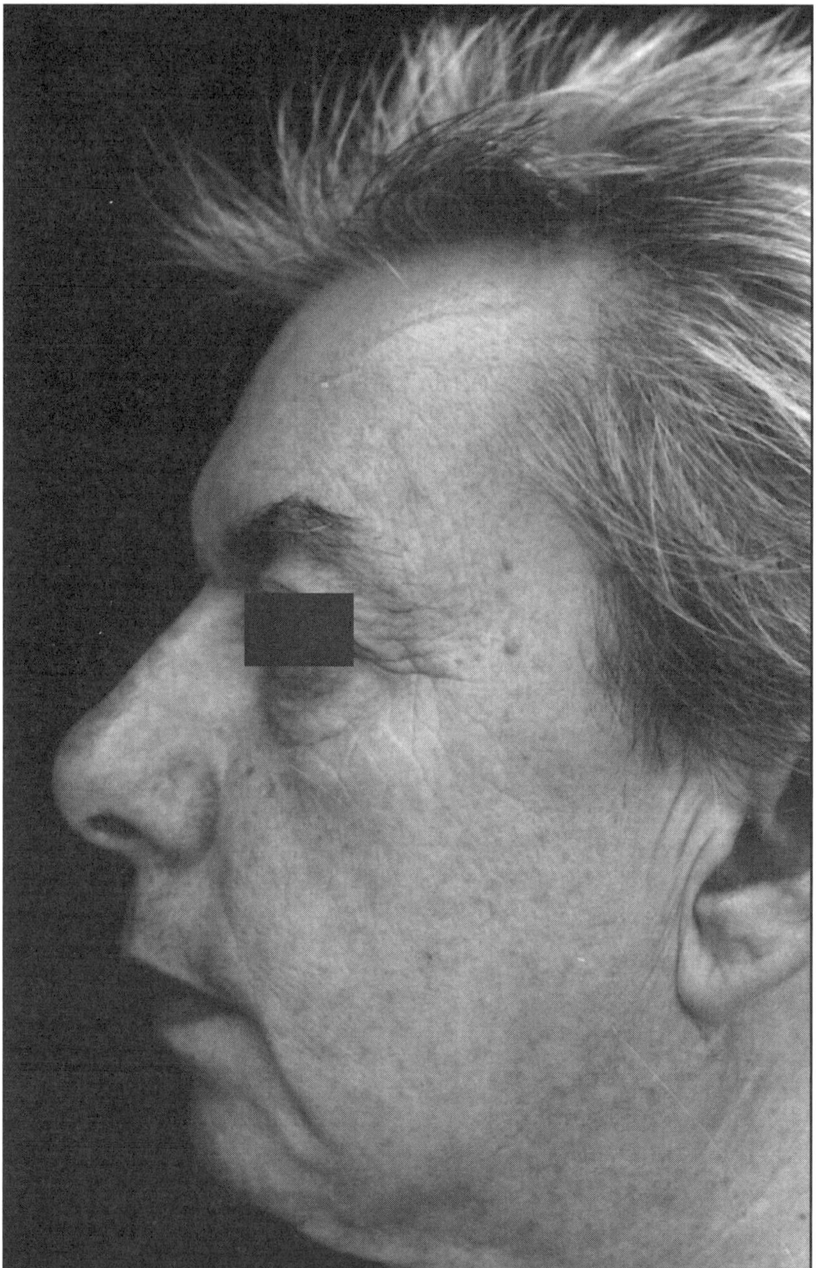

Before: chin weakness

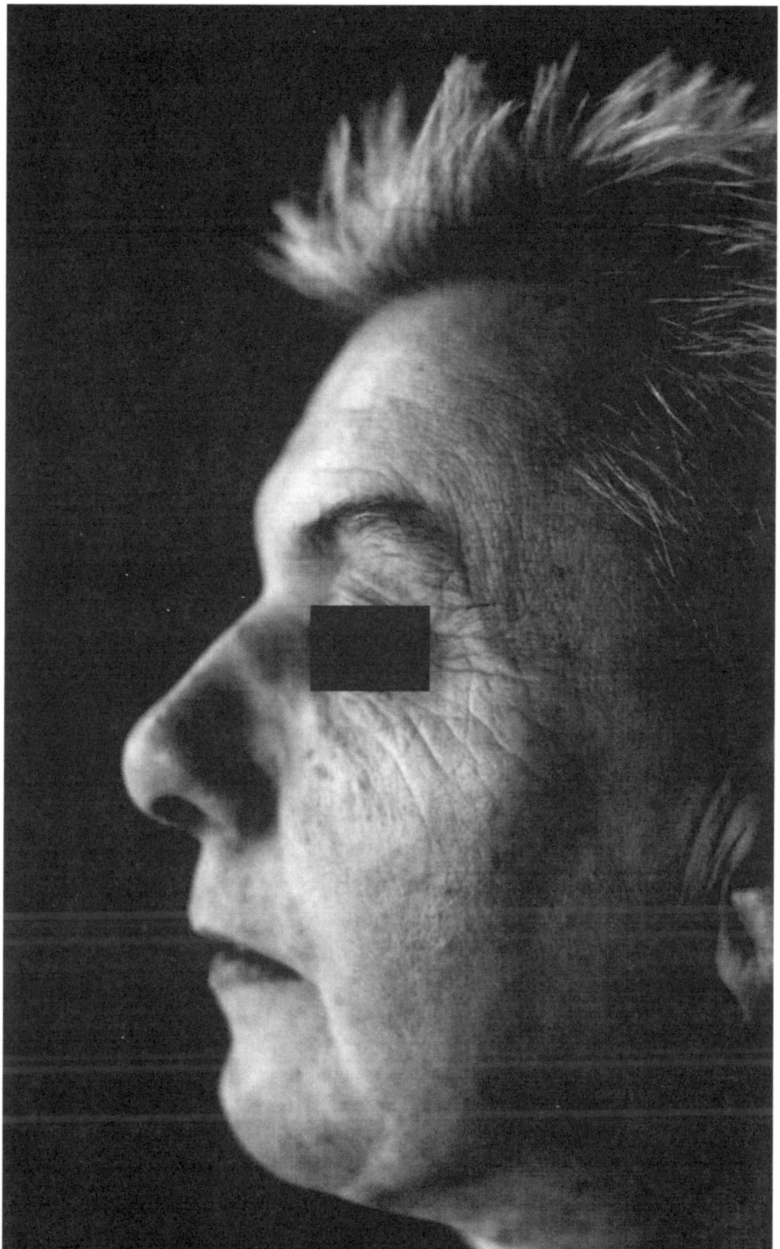

After chin correction with 12 c.c of permanent filler

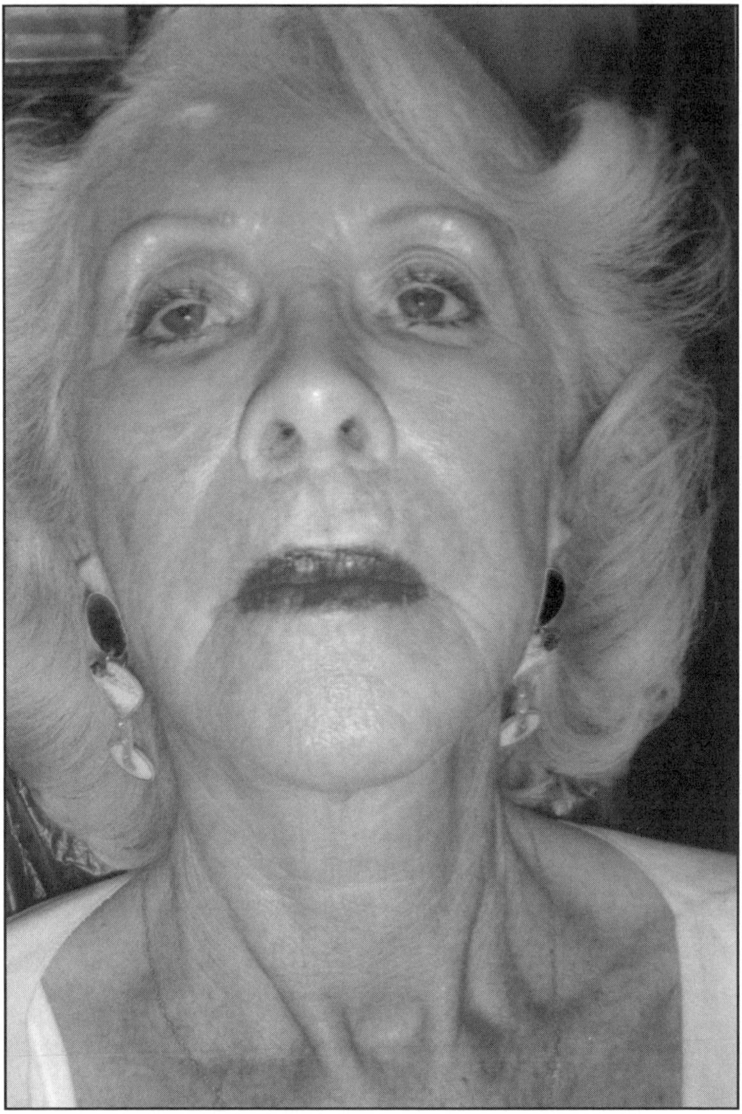

Before: Supra-clavicle and supra-sternum depressions

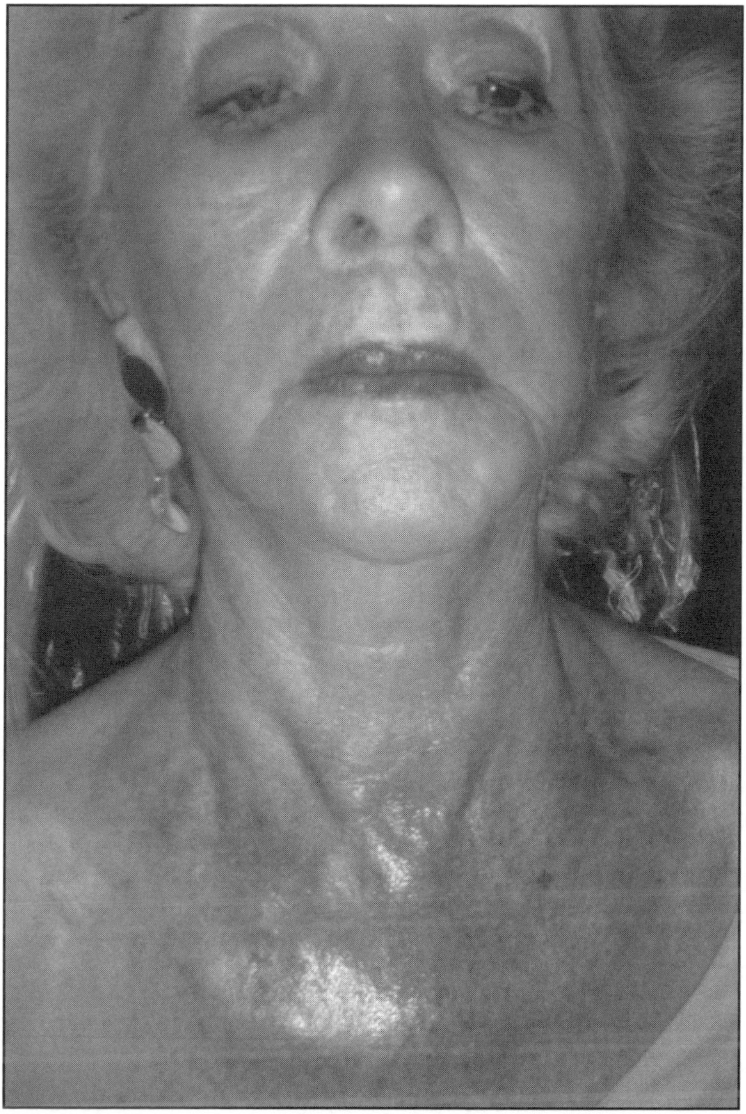

Supra-clavicle and supra-sternum treated with
120 c.c. of permanent filler.

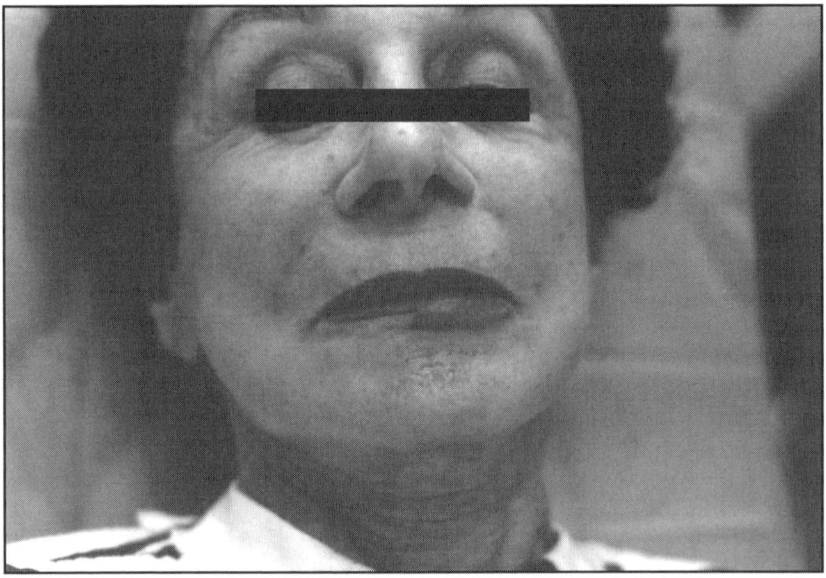

Lower lip correction. Notice that the photograph was taken after the injection of 1 c.c. of filler on her left side only.

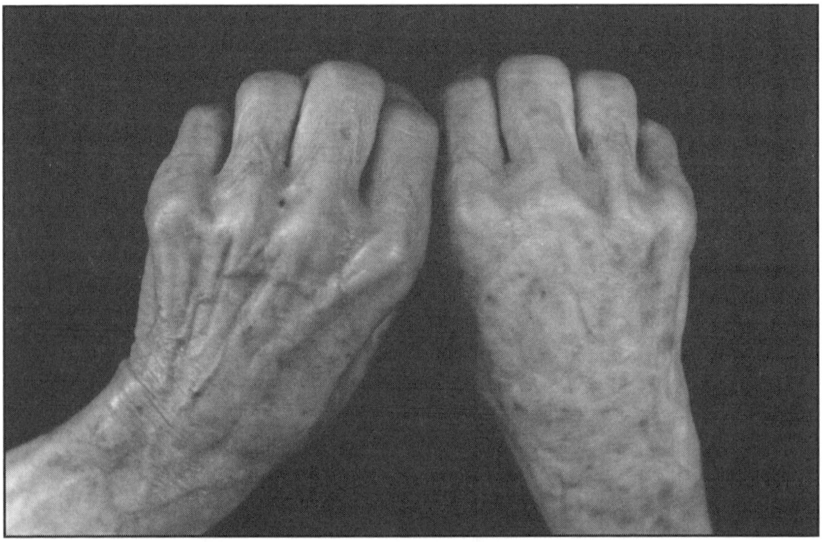

Back of hands before (left) and after (right) treatment with 20 c.c. of injectable filler

Back of Hands

A special section on the dorsum of the hands is necessary because as soon as we see your hands, we have a good idea of your age. With time the skin becomes very thin and the subcutaneous fat diminishes, producing "skeleton" effects, with the skin practically sitting on top of the tendons and muscles. In the United States, there are many cosmetic procedures for the face and neck, so there is a dramatic difference between faces and necks when compared with the hands. When women wear ostentatious rings or watches, instead of looking at the jewelry, we look at the depressions of the dorsum of the hands. My advice is if your hands do not look young any more, don't wear jewelry.

Our treatment for rejuvenating hands includes a special peel to remove hyperpigmentation, and we apply soft tissue fillers in an amount according to the depressions, between 1 or 2 c.c. per area. For many years we have followed this protocol with excellent permanent results.

Side Effects and Complications

Any soft-tissue filler, whether temporary or permanent, has some complications. The most common are edema, ecchymosis, erythema, discoloration, overcorrection due to excessive volume injected, "beading," and, in severe cases, granulomatous inflammatory reactions.

Despite these possible complications, the occurrence is extremely low; in the case of granulomas, one in seventy-five hundred cases.

Your doctor knows how to take care of these problems; he or she is a professional.

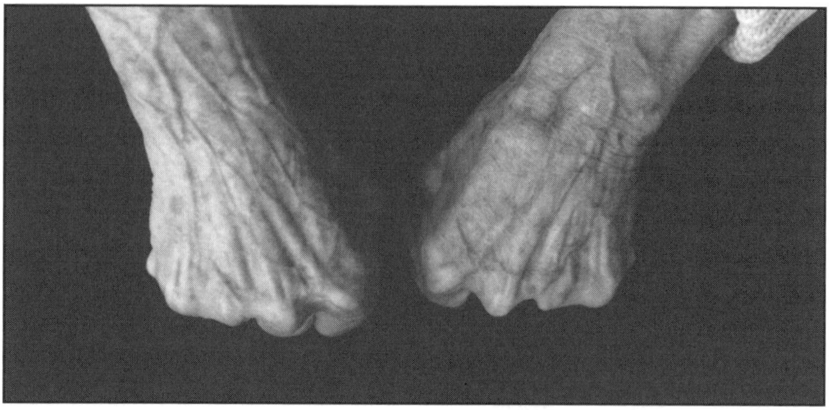

Hands before treatment

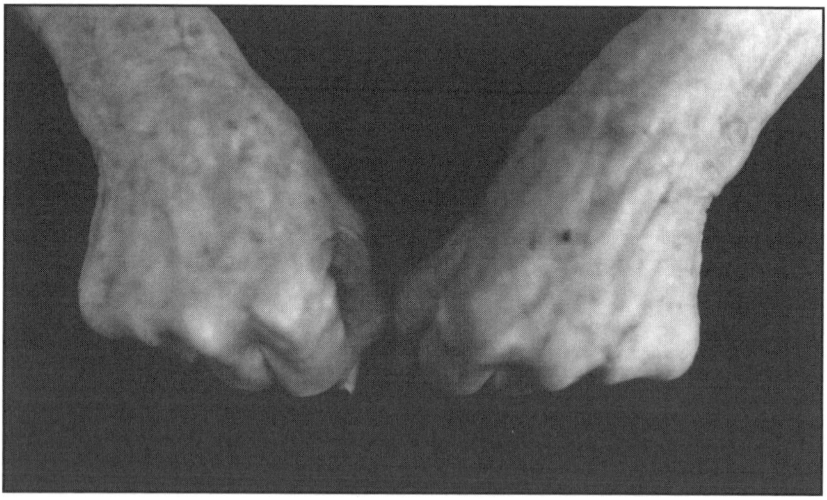

Hands after treatment with 22 c.c. of permanent filler

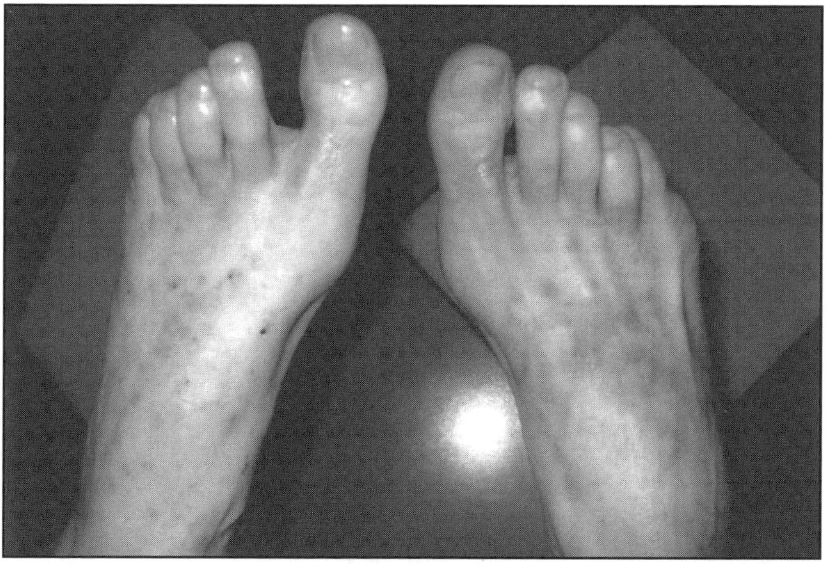

Injection of 10 c.c. of permanent filler (Right foot before treatment, left foot after treatment)

Further Reading

Ashley FI, Kees TD, Ballantyne DL Jr, Galloway D, Machica R, Grazer F, McConnell DV, Edgington T, and Kiskadden W. An injection technique for the treatment of facial hemiatrophy. *Plast & Reconstr Surg* 1965, 35, 64, 1965.

Ashley FI, Braley S, Rees, TD, Goulian D, and Ballantyne DI Jr. The present status of silicone fluid in soft tissue augmentation. *Plast & Reconstr Surg* 1967; 39:411.

Ashley FI, Braley S, and McNali, FG. The current status of silicone injection therapy. *Surg Clin N Am* 1971; 51:501.

Baker TC. Chemical face peeling and rhytidectomy. *Plast Reconstr Surg* 1962; 29:199

Baker TJ, Gordon HL. The ablation of rhytides by chemical means: a peliminary report. J Fla Med Assoc 1961; 48:451.

Ballantyne, DL Jr, Rees TD, and Seidman I. Silicone Fluids: response to massive subcutaneous injection of dimethylpolysiloxan fluid in animals. *Plast & Reconstr Surg* 1965; 36:330.

Balkin SW. Injectable silicone and the foot: a 41 year clinical and histologic history. *Dermatol Surg* 2005; 31:1555-1559.

Barnett JG, Barnett CR. Treatment of acne scars with liquid silicone injection: 30 years perspective. *Dermatol Surg* 2005; 31:(11 Pt 2): 1552-1549.

Bea-Hur N and Neuman Z: Siliconoma, another cutaneous reaction to silicone fluid. *Plast & Reconstr Surg* 1965; 36:629.

Blocksma R. Experience with dimethylpolysiloxane fluid in soft tissue augmetation. *Plast & Reconstr Surg* 1971, 48:564.

Brody HJ. Chemical peeling. St Louis: C.V. Mosby, 1997.

Brodland DJ, Roenigk RK. trichloroacetic acid chemexfoliation for extensive premalignant actinic damage of the face and scalp. Mayo Clin Proc 1988; 63:887.

Bryan CP. Ancient Egyptian medicine: the papyrus Ebers (translation). Chicago Ares Publishers, 1974:158-161.

Dingman DL, Hartog J, Siemionow M. Simultaneous deep-plane facelift and trichloroacetic acid peel. *Plast Reconstr Surg* 1994; 93:86-93.

Duffy DM. Liquid silicone for soft tissue augmentation. *Dermatol Surg* 2005; 31(11 pt2): 1530-1541 Review.

Ebbell B. Papyrus ebers (translation). Copenhagen: Ejmar Munksgaard,1937.

Fitzpatrick TB. The validity and practicality of sun-reactive skin types I-IV *Arch Dermatol* 1988; 124:869-871.

Gilles HD, Millard DR The principles and art of plastic surgery. Boston: Little Brown & Co., 1957:403.

Glogau RG Chemical peeling and aging skin. J *Geriat Dermatol* 1994; 2(1):30-35.

Goldman PM, Freed MI. Aesthetic problems in chemical peeling. J *Dermatol Surg Oncol* 1989; 15:1020-1024.

Grimes PE. Melasma-ideology and therapeutic considerations. *Arch Dermatol* 1995; 131:1453-1457.

Hexsel, DM, Hexsel CI, Iyengar V. Liquid injectable silicone: history, mechanism of action, indications, techniques and complications. Semin Cutan Med Sur 2003; 22(2):107-114. Review.

Jones D. HIV Facial lipoatrophy: causes and treatment options. *Dermatol Surg* 2005; 31(11pt2);1519-1529; discussion 1529. Review.

Litton C. Chemical face peeling. *Plast Reconstr Surg* 1962; 29:371.

MacKee GM, Karp FL. Treatment of post acne scars with phenol. Br J Dermatol 2953z; 64:456-459.

McCollough EG, Hillman RA. Chemical face peel Otolaryngol Clin North Am 1980; 13:353-365.

Mullison FG. Current status of silicone in plastic surgery. *Arch Otolaryng*, 1966; 83, 85.

Narins RS, Beer K. Liquid injectable silicone a review of history, immunology, technical considerations, complications, and potential. *Plast Reconstr Surg* 2006; 118(3 Suppl):778-845. Review.

Orentreich D. Liquid injectable silicone: techniques for soft tissue augmentation. *Clin Plast Surg* 2000; 28(4):595-612. Review.

Prather CI, Jones DH. Liquid injectable silicone for soft tissue augmentation. *Dermatol Ther* 206; 19(3):159-168.

Rees TD, and Ashley FL. Treatment of facial atrophy with liquid silicone. Am J Surg, 1966; 111:531.

Rohrich RJ, Potter JK. Liquid injectable silicone: is there a role as cosmtic soft-tissuer filler? *Plast Reconstr Surg* 2004; 113(4):1239=1241.

Rees TD, and Ashley FL. A new treatment for facial hemiatrophy in children by injection of dimethylpolysiloxane fluid. *J Ped Surg* 1967; 2:347.

Roenigk RK. A primer of facial chemical peel. Dermatol Clin 1993; 11(2):349-359.

Sanchez PH, et al. Melasma. J *Am Acad Dermatol* 1981; 4:68-710.

Symmers, C. Silicone mastitis in "topless" waitress and some other varieties of foreign body mastitis. *Brit Med J* 1968; 3:19.

Urkov JC. Surface defects of skin: treatment by controlled exfoliation. Ill Med J 1946; 89:75.

Zappi E, Barnett JG, Zappi M, Barnett CR. The long-term host response to liquid silicone injected during soft tissue augmentation procedures: a microscopic appraisal. *Dermatol Surg* 2007; 33 Suppl2:S186-192; discussion 5192.

Chapter 4
Lifters (Soft Tissue)

As I mentioned, the future and main objective of modern cosmetic medicine is based upon a minimally invasive facial and corporal approach. This means minimal recuperation time and minimal expense for patients that, at age thirty-five, start to worry about their physical appearance. Our new generations do know that prevention is better. Because of this new phenomenon, our industry is producing more peelers, lifters, and soft tissue fillers.

Russian and Brazilian "Threads"

Soft tissue "lifters" were created by a team of Russian doctors (father and son) Marlen and George Sulamanidze. In our clinic, we use the Brazilian version designed by Dr. José Beramendi in Rio de Janeiro. These threads are made of polypropylene, a material widely used in general surgery as nonabsorbable suture material. The threads can go from 1 to 5mm in thickness and several centimeters in length. The edges have "spikes" or "teeth" in convergent directions that, once they have been attached to the inside of the skin, provide the "lifting" effect with autostability.

We call it a nonsurgical face-lift whose main advantages are:

1) It is a minimally invasive procedure.
2) It can be performed at a doctor's office.
3) It is done under local anesthesia.
4) The results are equivalent to a mini-surgery
5) There are no scars or stitches to remove.

Procedure

The treatment is done under local anesthesia in the doctor's office, with the aid of a 10-15 cm cannula that is inserted under the skin and exits from the lower part of the face. The cannula produces a tunnel though which the thread is inserted. Once the threads enter and exit, the cannula is removed, and the threads are anchored in the posterior part of the skin. Then the operator manually pulls up the skin and the top part of the thread is attached to the capsule of the termporal muscle. The nonsurgical face-lift provides a soft tissue lifting effect, diminishing the wrinkled tissues.

This procedure is recommended for:

1) Tail of the eyebrows
2) Middle part of the face
3) Skin of the jawline
4) Upper part of the neck

It is important to add that the "threads" cannot be absorbed by the body, so the tendency is to encapsulate them the same way that nonabsorbable, injectable materials are encapsulated. This reaction favors augmentation of the volume of the face.

Results

As you can appreciate from the following photographs, after two to three months, the clinical effect of a nonsurgical face-lift is very interesting and rewarding both for patient and doctor. This is a good alternative to plastic surgery.

It is important to add that the proper selection of viable patients, proper planning, and proper thread insertion under sterile conditions are what produce the good results.

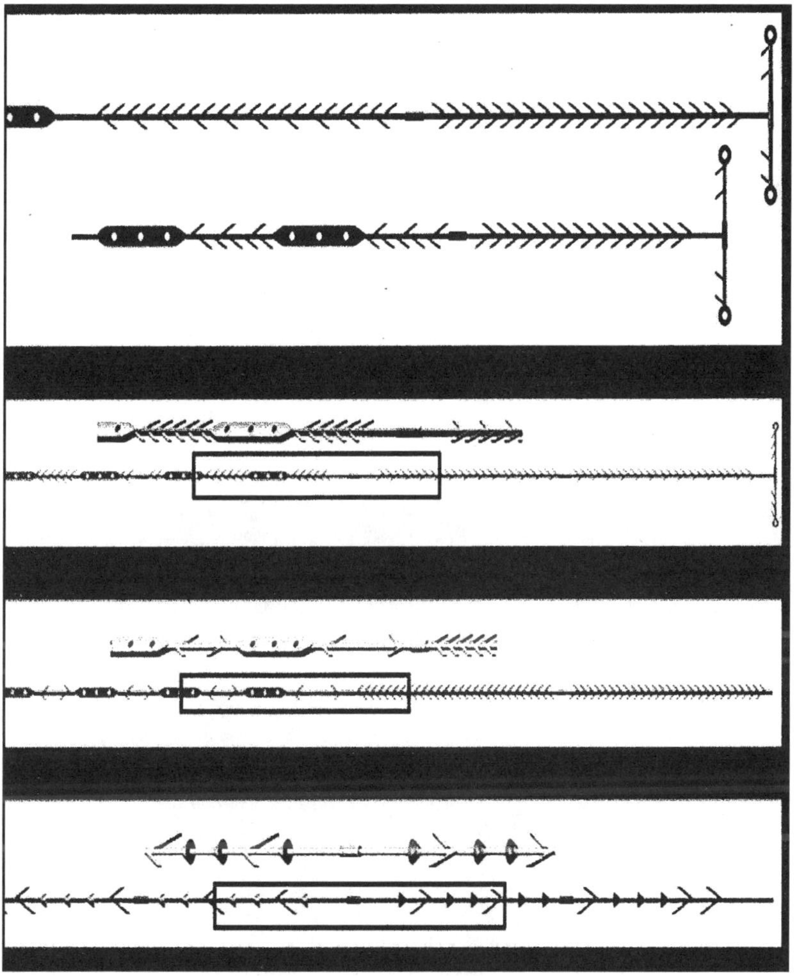

Different types of Brazilian "threads"

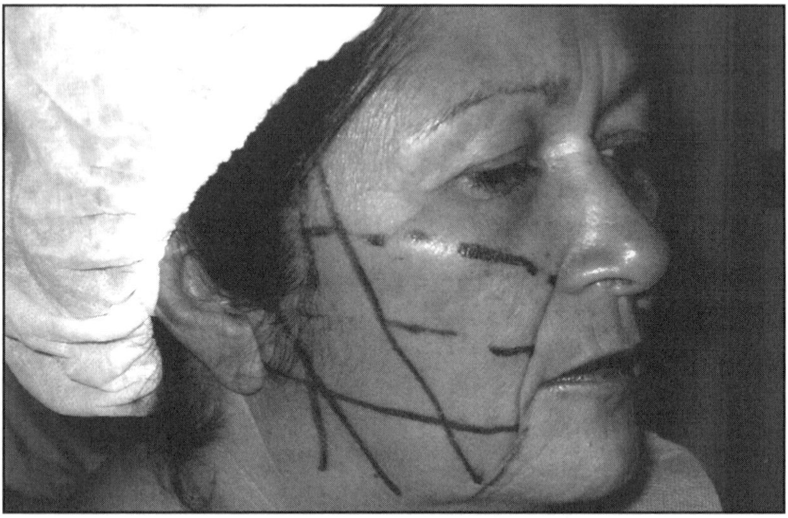

Facial markings before Brazilian "threads."

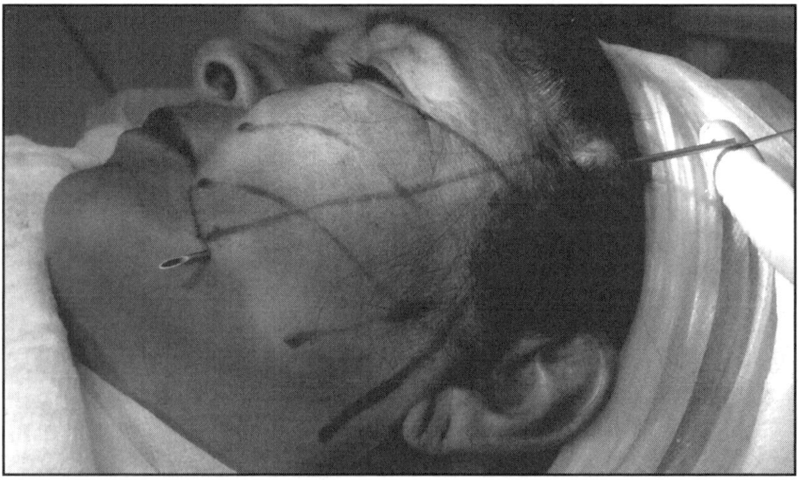

The cannula produces a tunnel for the "threads."

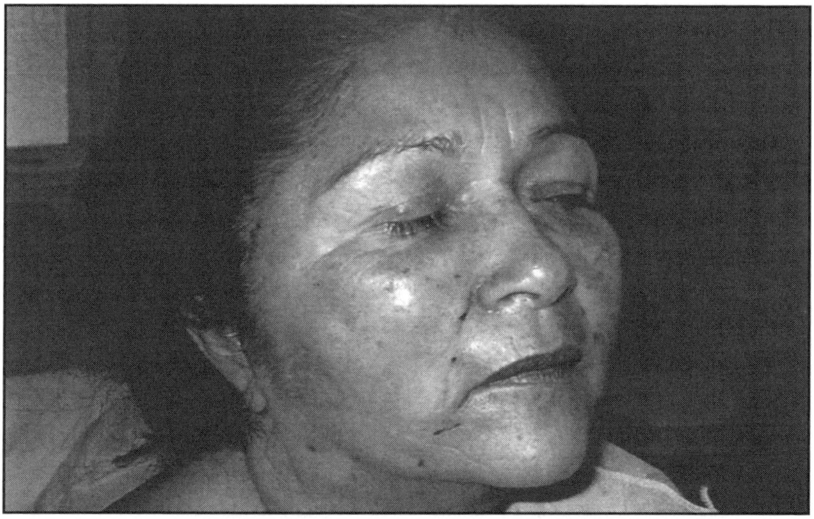

Immediately after full procedure.
Note the complete absence of swelling.

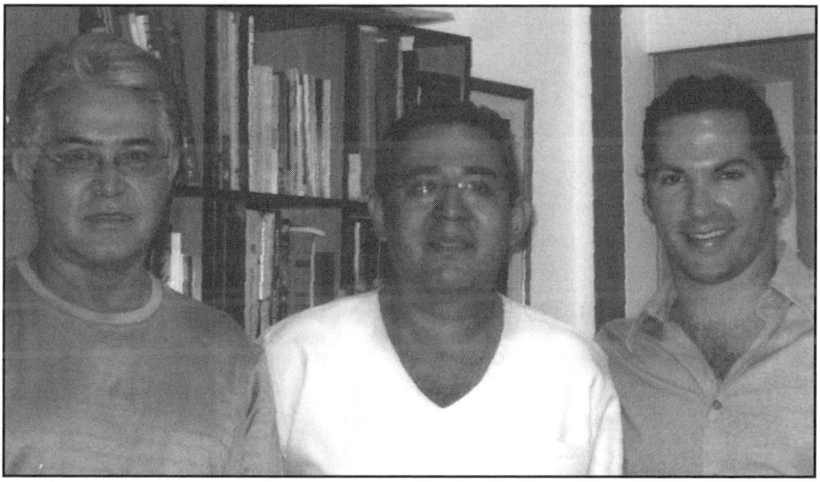

Doctors Carlos Soria (L) and Karlo Soria (R) with Dr. Beramendi in Rio de Janeiro.

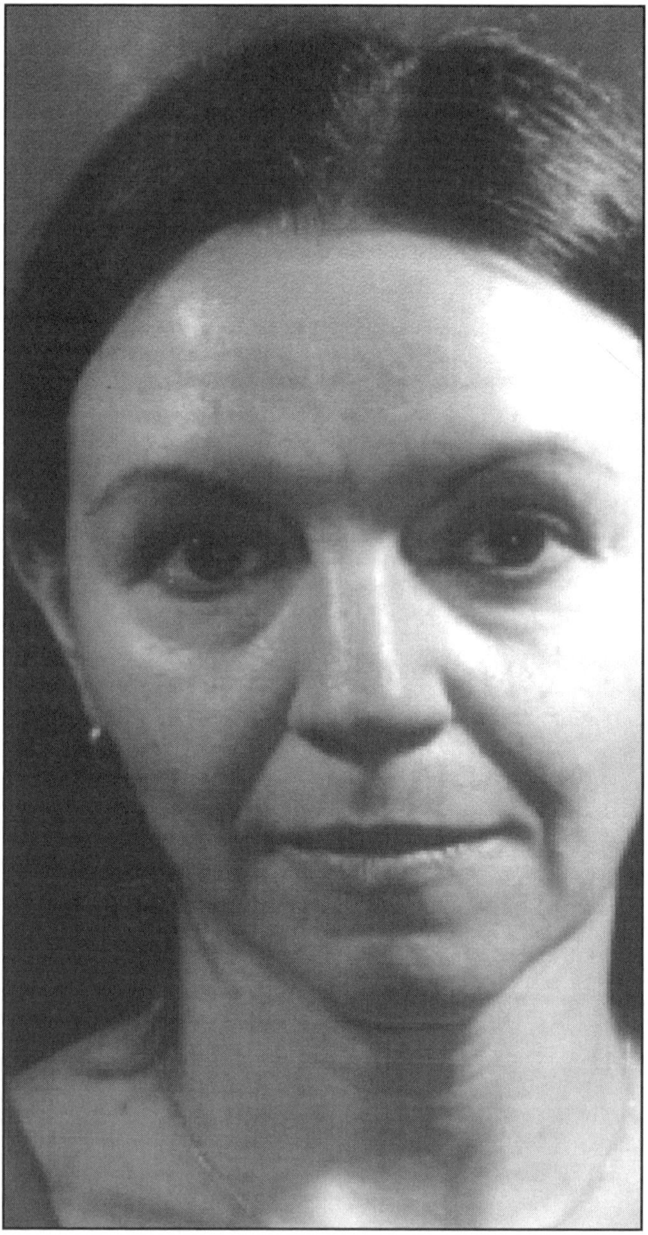

A 37-year-old patient with light gravitational effect on side of face; notice nasolabial folds.

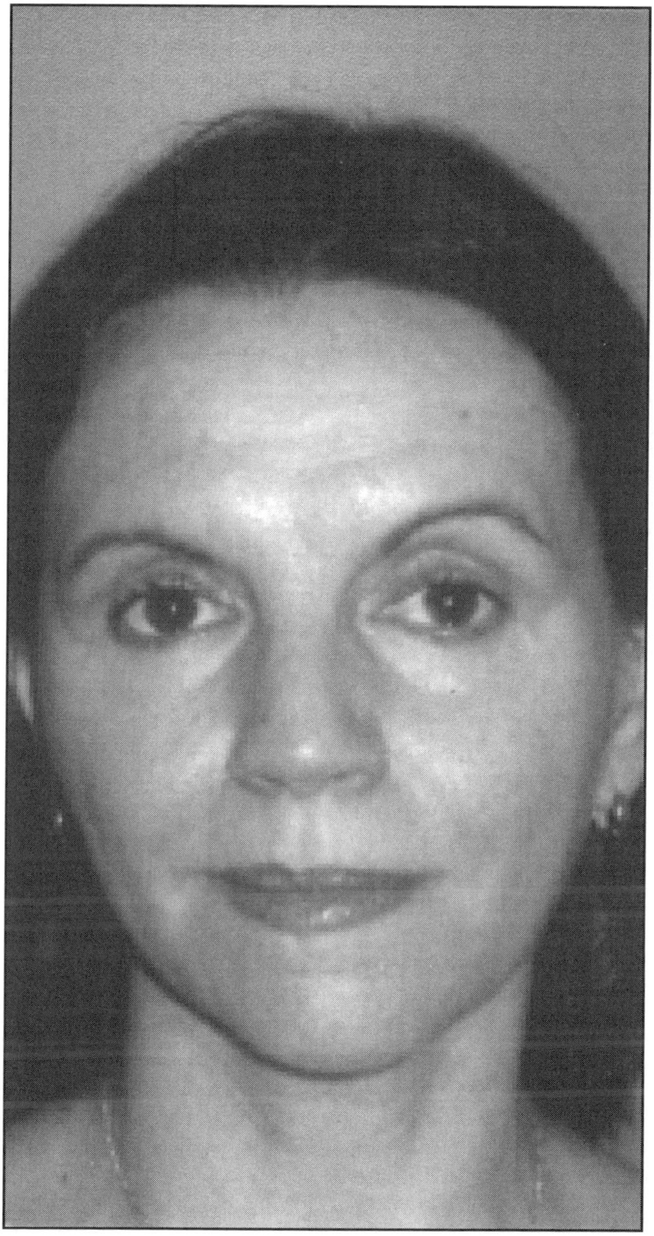

Same patient three months after placement of 5 "threads" in each side of the face.

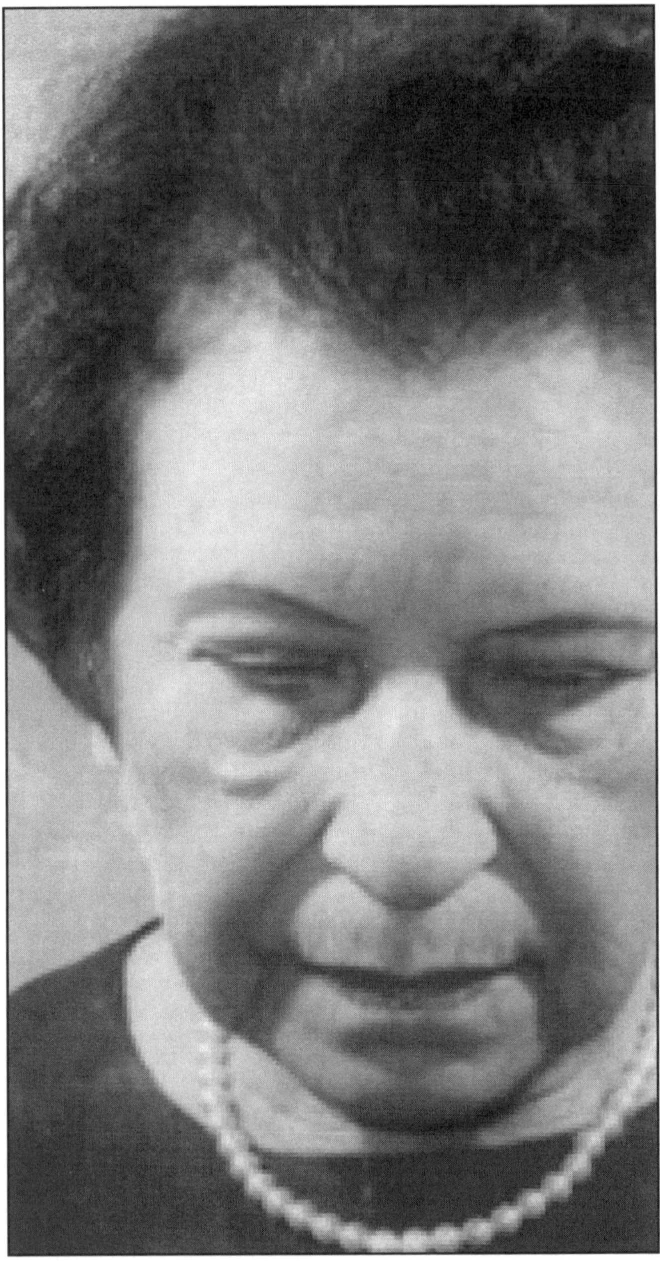

A 74-year-old patient with severe facial folds.

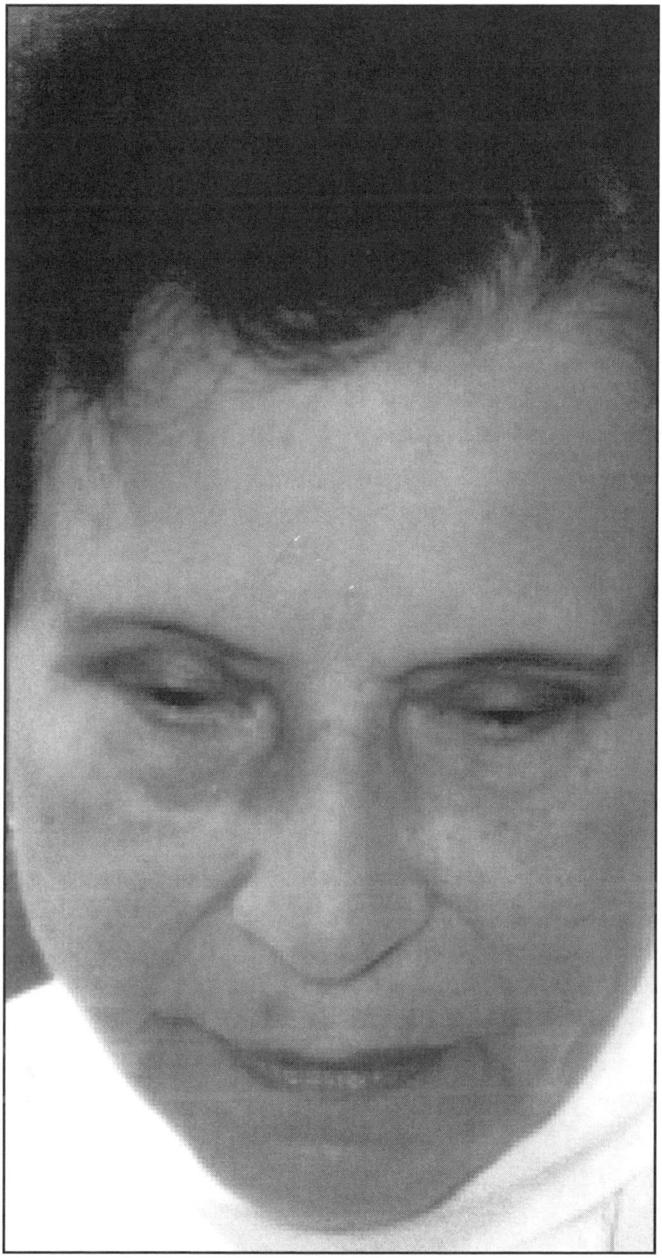

Same patient six months after the insertion of eleven Brazilian threads on each side of the face.

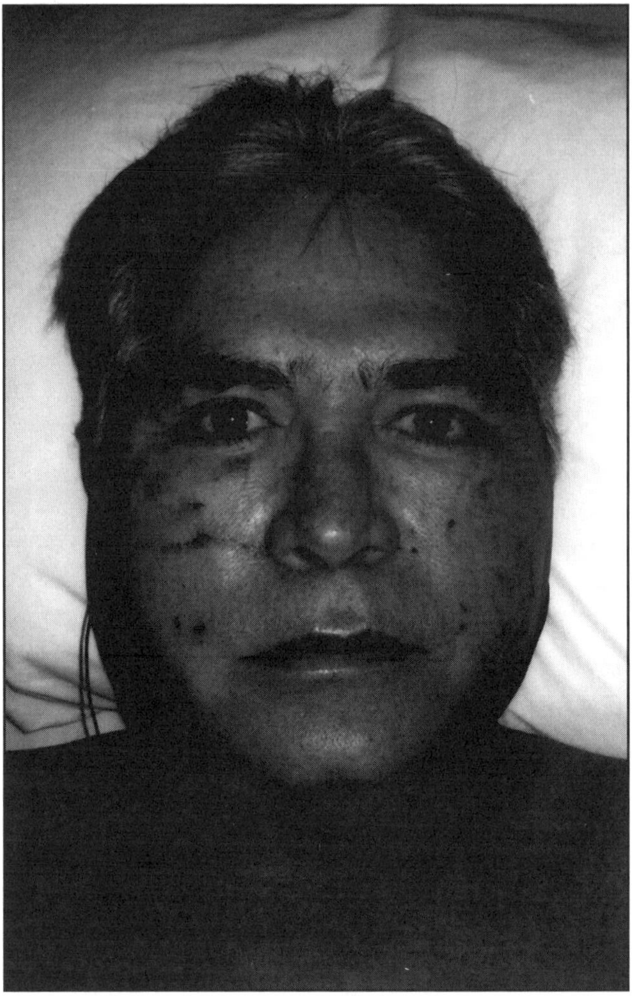

Dr. Carlos Soria's face immediately after Brazilian lifts with Dr. Veramendi's threads.

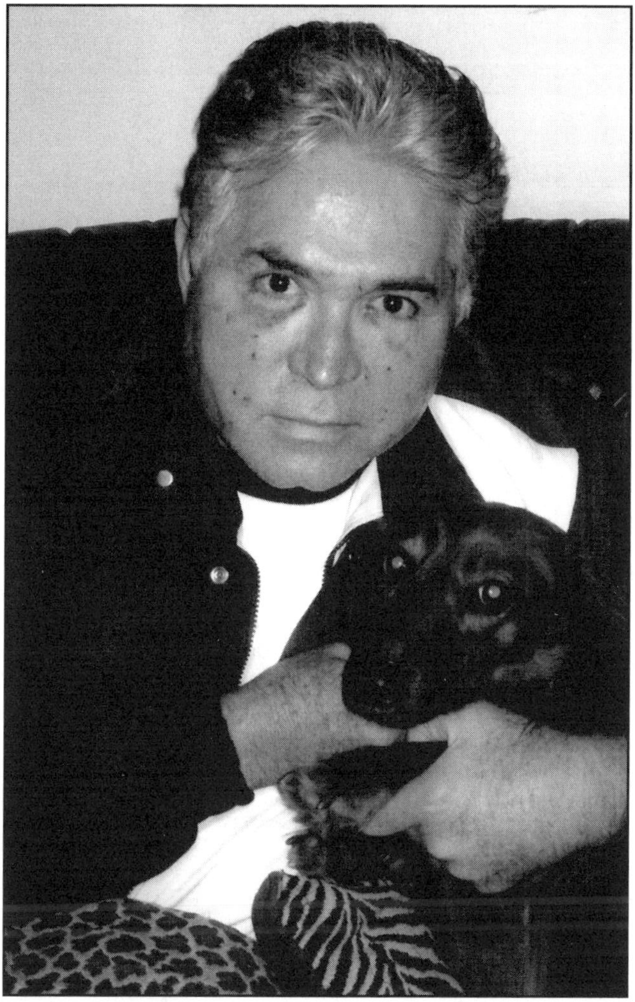

The following day with Doctor's "Chicha."

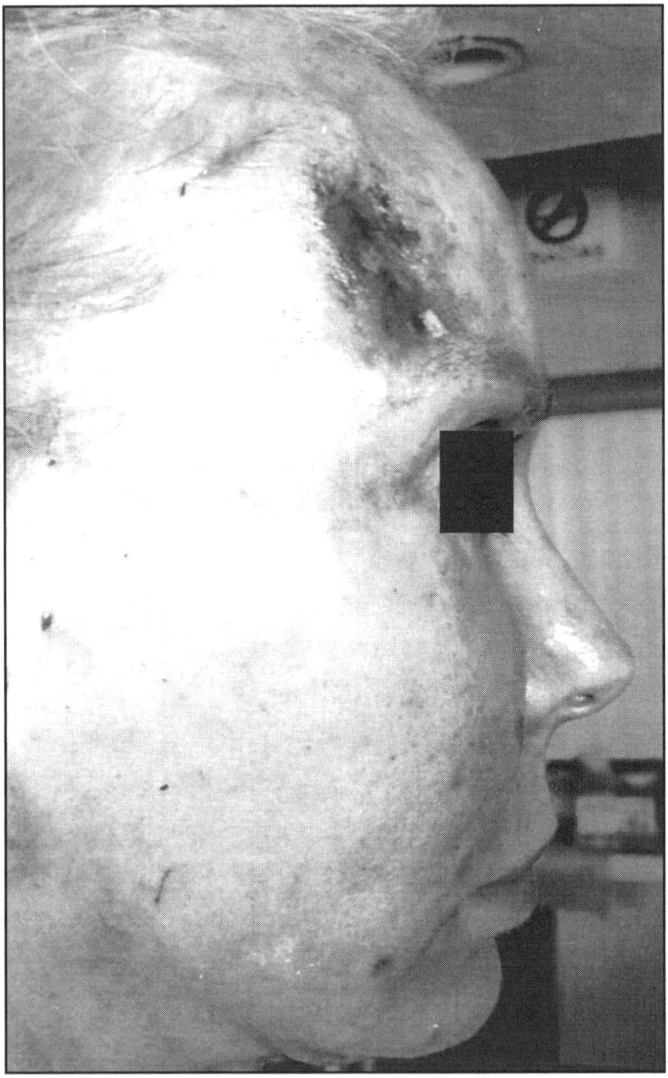

Frontal infection resolved with antibiotics after 2 weeks

Further Reading

Adamyan, AA et al. Clinical aspects of facial skin reinforcement with special (gold) surgical filaments. *Ann of Plast Rec and Aest Surg* 1009; 3:18-22.

De la Plaza R, Arroyo JM. A new technique for the treatment of palpebral bags. *Plast Reconstr Surg* 1988; 102:1646-1657.

Freeman MS. Transconjunctival Suv-Orbicularis Oculi Fat (SOOF) Pad Lift Blepharoplasty, *Arch Facial Plast Surg* 2000; Vol 2, Jan-Mar.

Hamra ST. The zygorbicular dissection in composite rhtidectomy: an ideal midface plane. Plast Reconstr Surg 1998: 102:1646-1657.

Kazinnikova, OG, Adamian AA. Age-specific changes in facial and cervical tissues. A review. *Ann of Plast Rec and Aest Surg* 2000; 1:52-61.

Mitz V, Peironye M. The superficial musculo-aponeurotic system in the parotid and cheek area. *Plast Reconstr Surg* 12976; 58, 80.

Owsley JQ. Lifting the malar fat pad correction of prominent nasolabial folds. *Plast Reconstr Surg* 1993; 91:463-474.

Skoog T. Plastic Surgery, New Methods and refinements. Almquist and Wiksell International, Stockholm, 1974, 301-303.

Sulmanidze MA, et al. Flabby, ageing face. A new approach. World Congress on Aesthetic and Restorative Surgery, Mumbai, February 2001. 54.

Sulamanidze MA, et al. Wire Scalpel for Surgical Correction of Soft Tissue Contour Defects by Subcutaneous Dissection. *Dermatol Surg* 2001 Feb; 26(2):146-151.

Chapter 5
Body Augmentation

One of the most fascinating aspects of medical aesthetics is without a doubt the "revolutionary" approach to body augmentation in areas like the buttocks, arms, pectorals, and legs. These procedures were designed by Dr. Almir Moojen Nácul in Brazil.

But before going into body augmentation, let me tell you that this has been a controversial topic since the1950s. Many in Hollywood and Las Vegas have been injected with large volumes of liquid silicone, especially in breasts and buttocks. Not only was body augmentation practiced in America, but in Japan at that time, prostitutes were injected to "look more American," to appeal to American servicemen based in Japan.

Not only silicone, but paraffin, Vaseline, and other oils—like baby oil—were utilized, as in the famous Dr. Sakurai formula. A few years later, Dr. Sakurai moved to Beverly Hills in California to work with his relatives.

All these techniques were prior to the invention of breast implants filled with silicone, which were controversial as well (in the United States). Patients' lawyers sued doctors and breast implant manufacturers with allegations that those implants produced "arthritis-like conditions" in patients after being implanted! Finally, after multiple studies done all over the world, the scientific community ruled that there was no connection between silicone breast implants and autoimmune diseases (arthritis).

Today, the commercial use of plastic bags containing silicone for breast augmentation is common the world over, and it's business as usual.

In 2008, I had the opportunity to travel to Porto Alegre in Brazil and meet Dr. Almir Moojen Nácul, plastic surgeon, designer, and promoter of bioplasty. Since then I have followed his protocol and used his material under the name of New Plastic (PMMA), polymethyl methacrylate, which consists of microspheres of plastic, just like the material they use to manufacture contact lenses. These microspheres are suspended in a non-protein gel and come in concentrations of 2 to 10 and 30 percent.

Facial and corporal bioplasty with bio-implants is performed by injecting intramuscularly by means of cannulas, respecting the corresponding different anatomical planes.

Everything starts with a consultation, a proper marking—planning on top of the skin of the patient, photographs, cleaning of the area, local injection of anesthesia (Xylocaine 2%), and finally by cannulas, the selected implant material is "accommodated" intramuscularly by means of honeycomb-like multiple tunnels.

All these procedures may take from 15 minutes to four hours and are done under local anesthesia that means that during the entire procedure, the patient is awake and gives her opinion about the results via talking with the doctor. Remember that during most plastic surgery procedures, the patient is under general anesthesia and has no opinion.

In bioplasty, we can inject an area and the patient can get up from the table, look in the mirror, and ask for more augmentation if he or she desires to do so.

Most patients do have a clear idea of the results they expect, for example, 50 percent more gluteal area. Although there are several surgical techniques for these purposes, bioplasty is the less invasive and has the fastest recuperation period.

The volumes to implant can vary from 1 to 4 c.c. to as much as 150 to 200 c.c. per session. After three months, we can add more volume if necessary. This is an ideal procedure to augment the projection of profile of the gluteal region or any muscle of the body.

Procedure

As we had mentioned, each procedure should be done under the strictest cleanliness guidelines. Conditions, if not sterile, should at least consist of a very clean consulting room, which will prevent as few complications as possible.

You and your treating physician should talk about the material that will be used and the areas to treat. A medical history should be done, and clinical photographs will be taken. Anesthesia is performed in its three variations: topical, infiltration, and nerve blocks. Your doctor should determine the amounts and types of anesthesia and the volume and concentration of the different fillers.

Complications and Secondary Effects

It is important to say that after more than thirty-five years of practice, I find that the results, although satisfactory, do carry very minimum side effects. In general, complications may be early or late. Early complications include edema, bruising, or inflammation of the injected site, temporary situations that can take from hours to a few days to resolve by themselves. This happens usually when the patient takes anticoagulants, aspirin, or multivitamins. The use of Arnica Montana as a homeopathic remedy is advisable.

Problems such as infections or "necrosis" (loss of tissue) are extremely rare; perhaps the most frequent complication is "over encapsulation," which feels like a bump after thirty to sixty days; it is easily corrected with a few drops of cortisone.

The different materials can be injected superficially in the dermis or very deep in the muscle. They can be done with needles or cannulas. It is your doctor and his or her experience that makes the difference. Dr. Nácul calls his technique "remodeling by bio-materials." We become sculptors, and your face or body is our marble. In our clinic, the favorite permanent materials are Dermagen and New Plastic. Both are permanent because the body, instead of destroying the material, encapsulates it within the next thirty to sixty days after the implantation.

Results

Since a photograph is better than a thousand words, please see the following results obtained in our clinic with the above mentioned material and techniques.

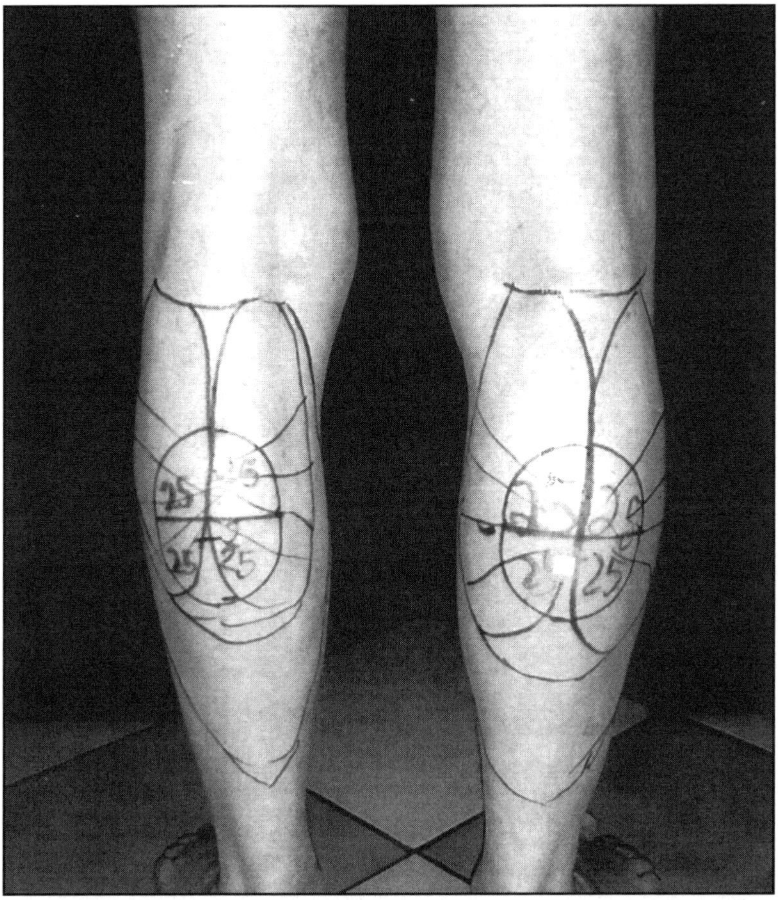

Designed calf augmentation; patient's left calf (on right) has been injected with 100 c.c. of permanent filler.

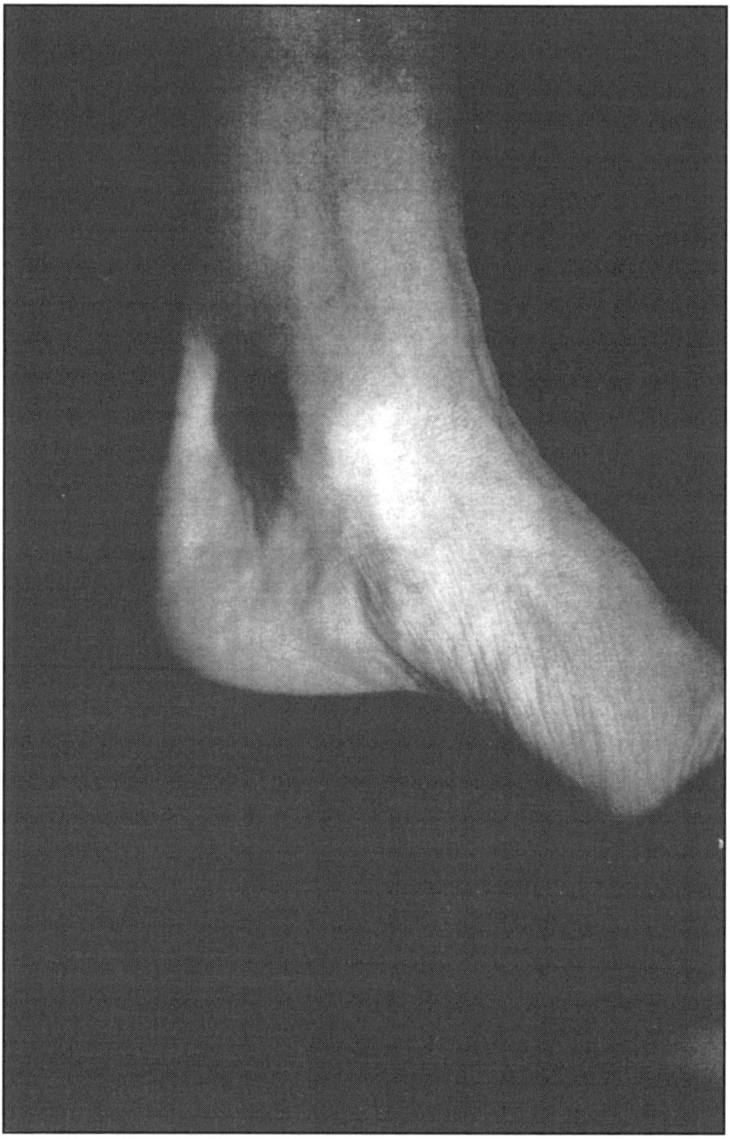

Significant depression on the inside of the left ankle.

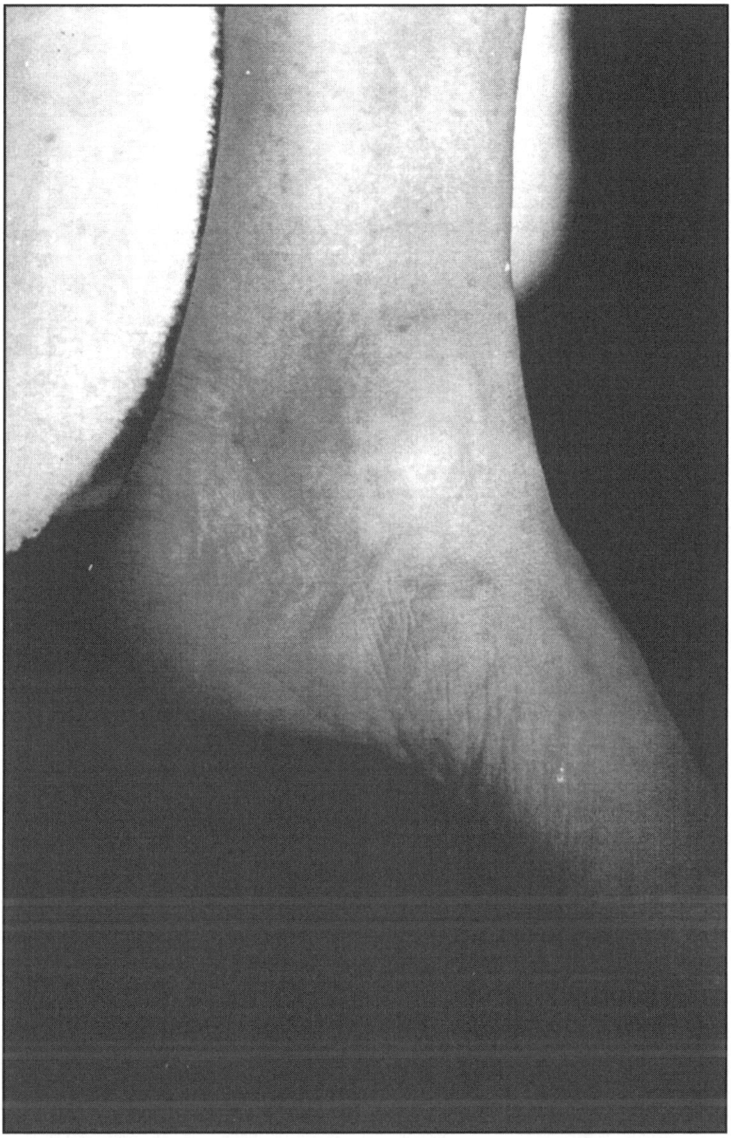

Internal area of the ankle treated with 50 c.c. of permanent filler.

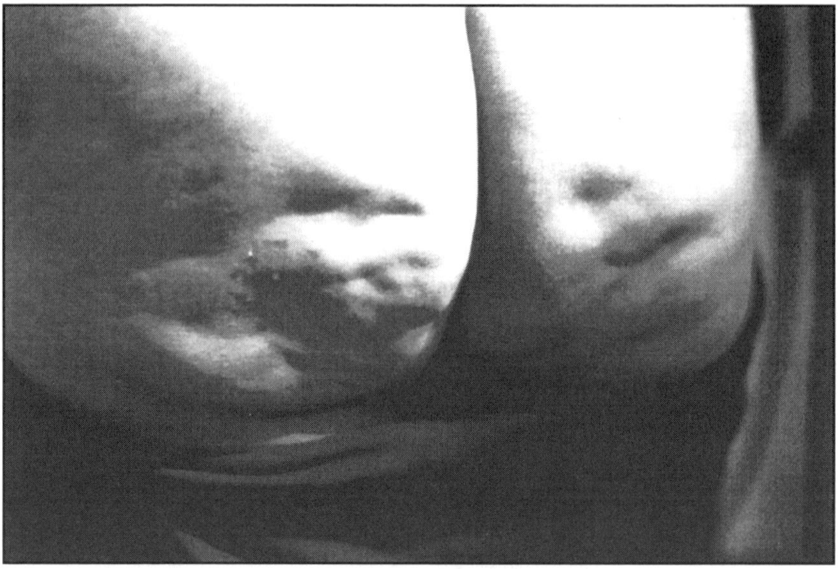

Before buttocks reconstruction.

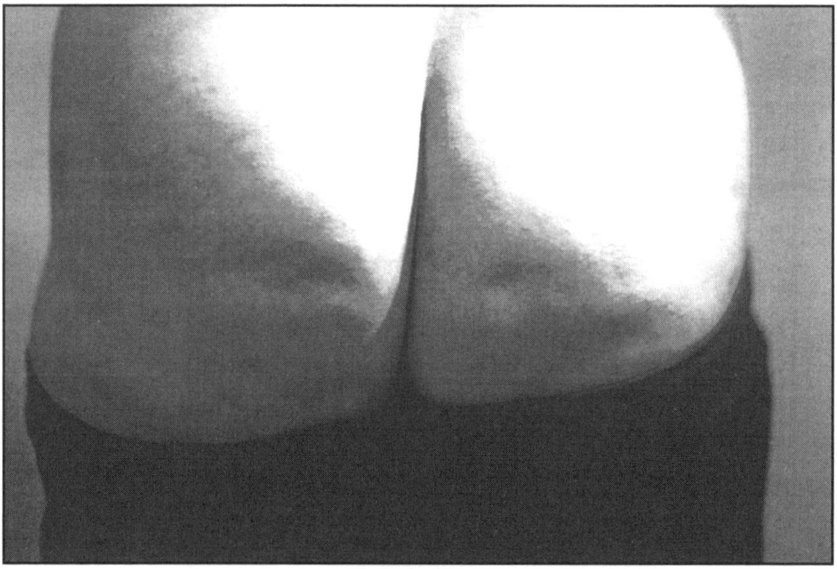

15 days after buttocks reconstruction with
250 c.c. of permanent filler.

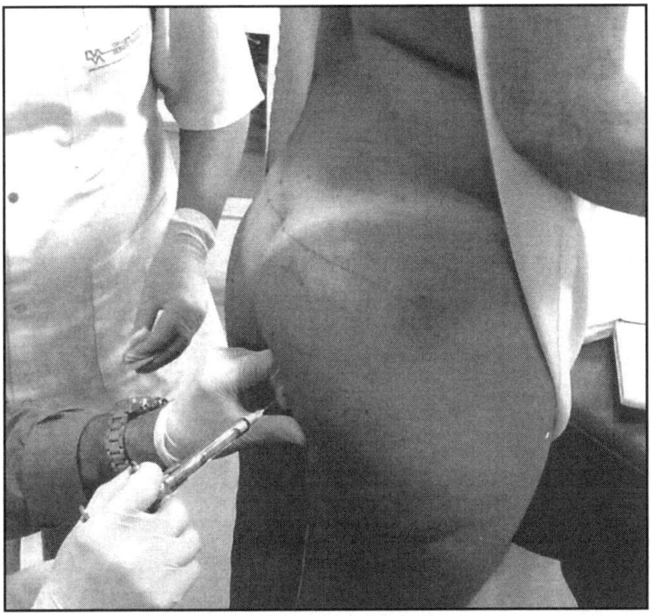

Gluteal enhancement with “New Plastic” in Brazil.

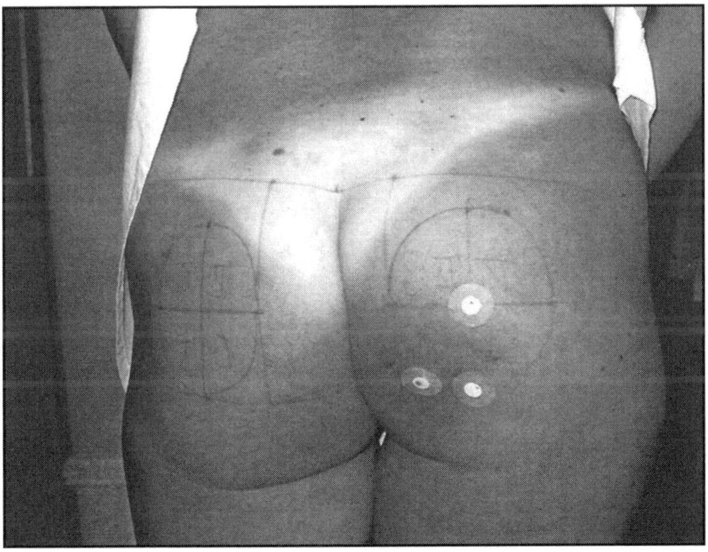

Left buttock designed but not done;
right buttock augmented with 150 c.c. of permanent filler.

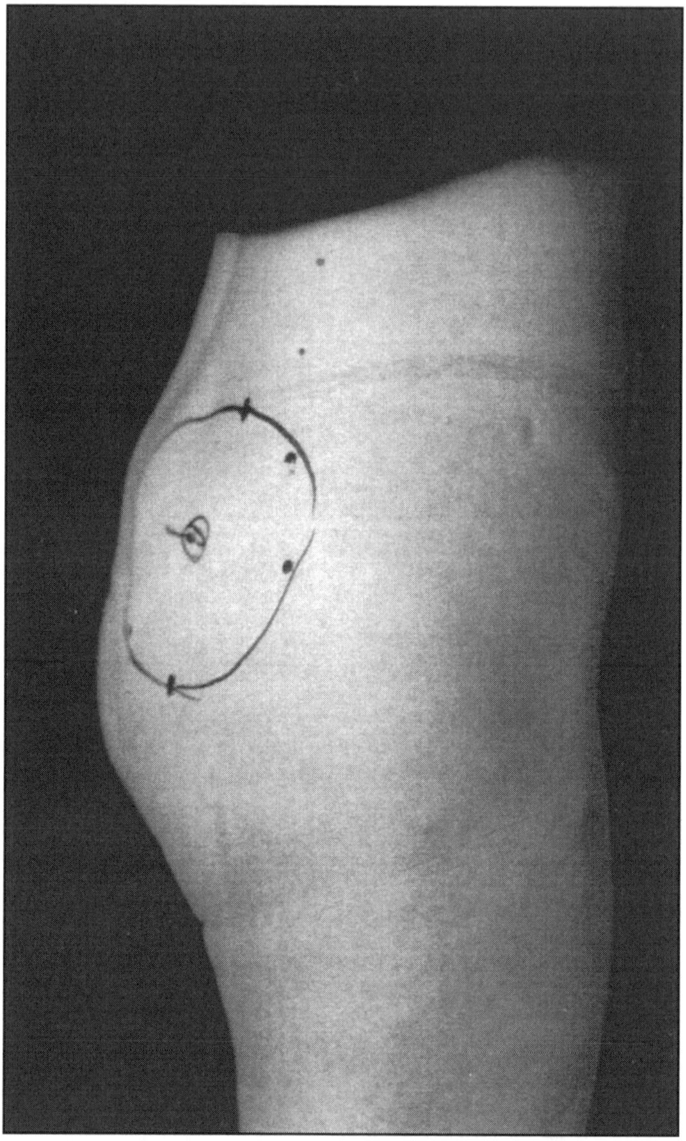

Buttocks augmentation, designed but not done.

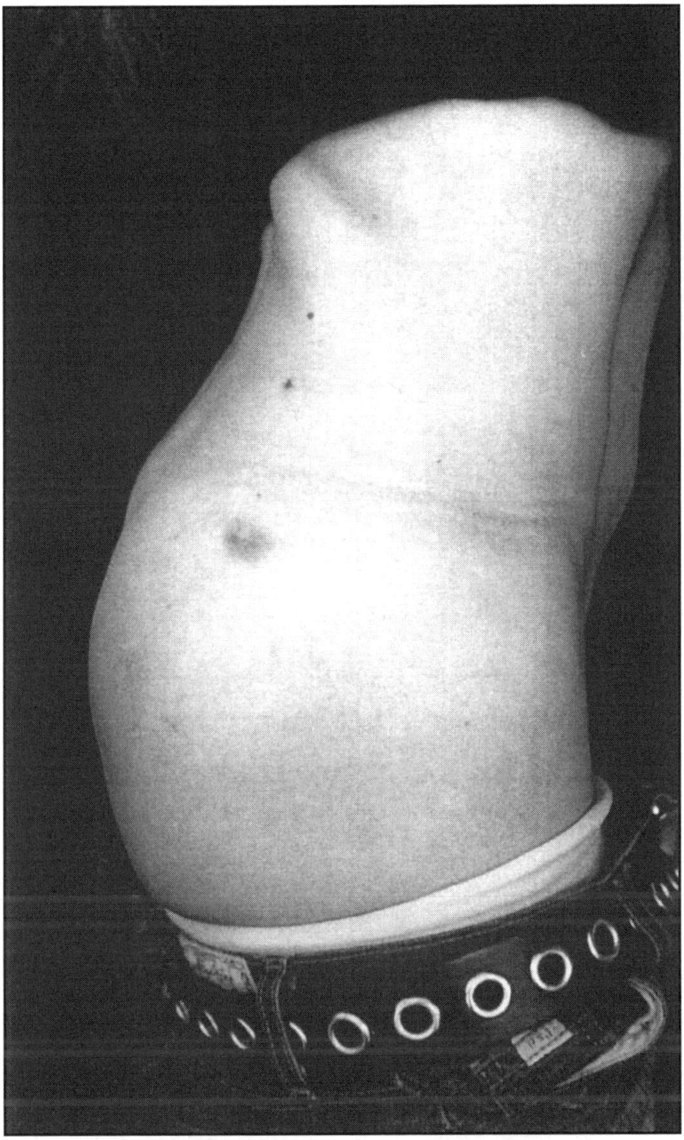

Results of buttocks augmentation with 250 c.c.
of permanent filler on each side

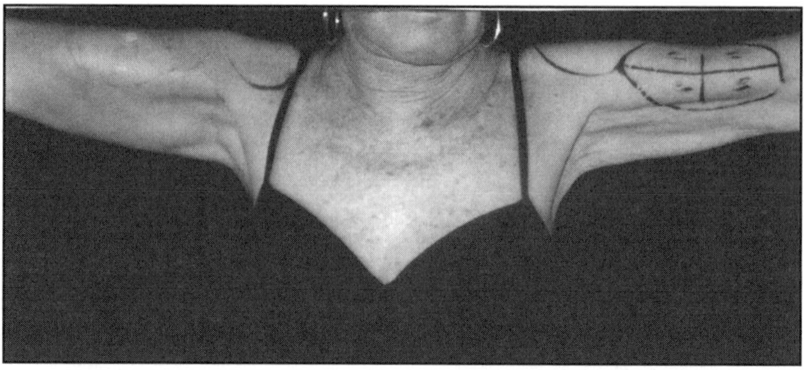

Upper arm augmentation before (on right) and after (on left) injection of permanent filler.

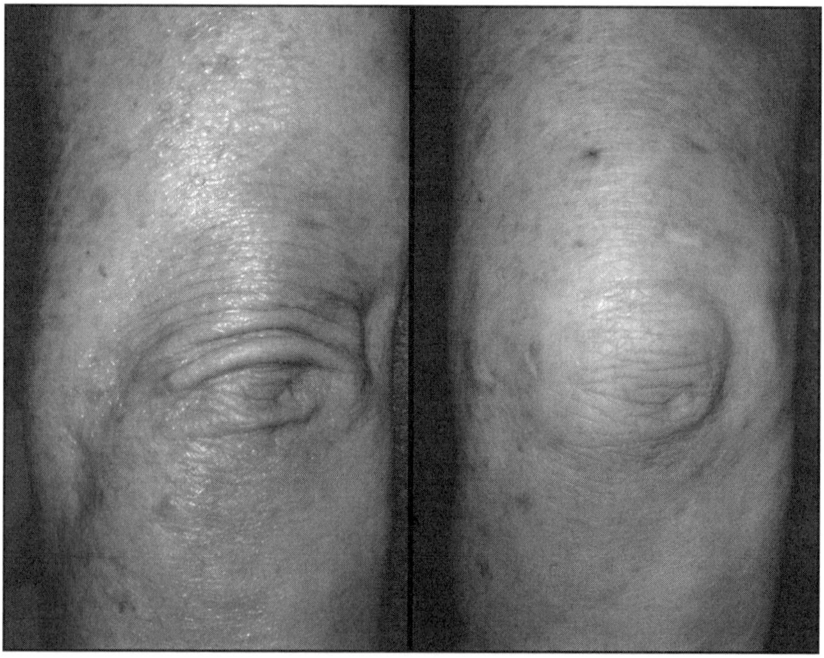

Before (left) and 6 months after after (right) injection of 25 c.c. of permanent filler into redundant elbow skin on a 55-year-old patient.

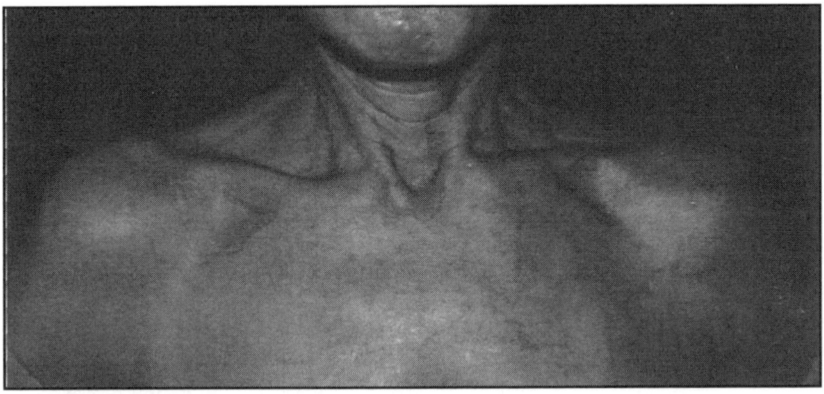

A 65-year-old patient with redundant skin and depression of supraclavicle sternum and chest areas before treatment.

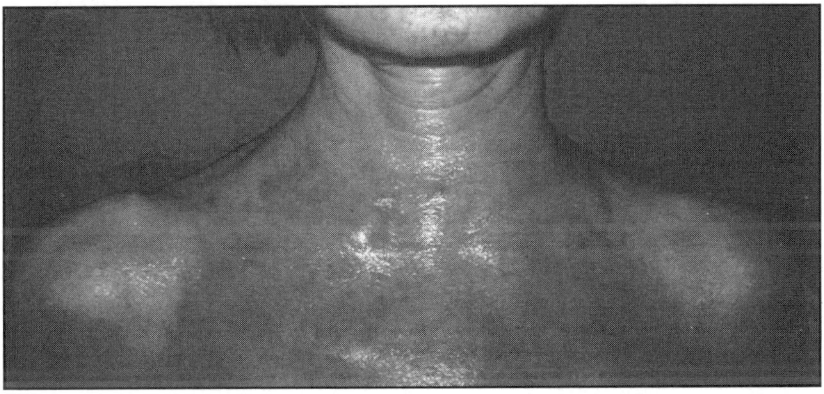

After treatment with 125 c.c. of permanent filler.

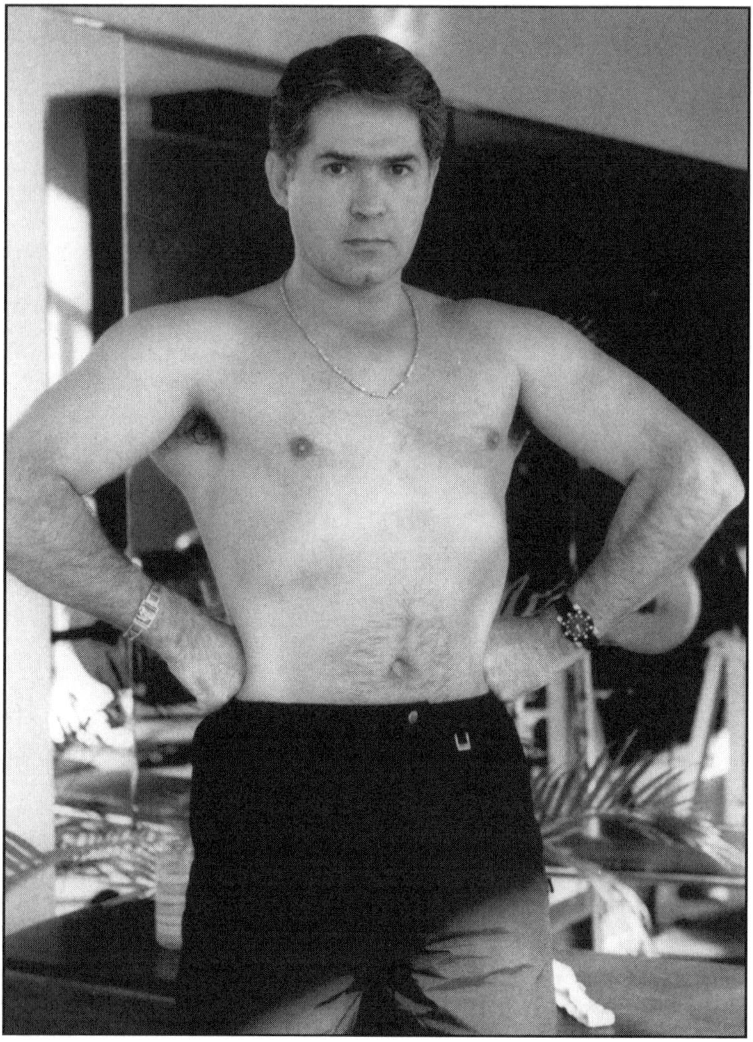

Dr. Carlos Soria at 35

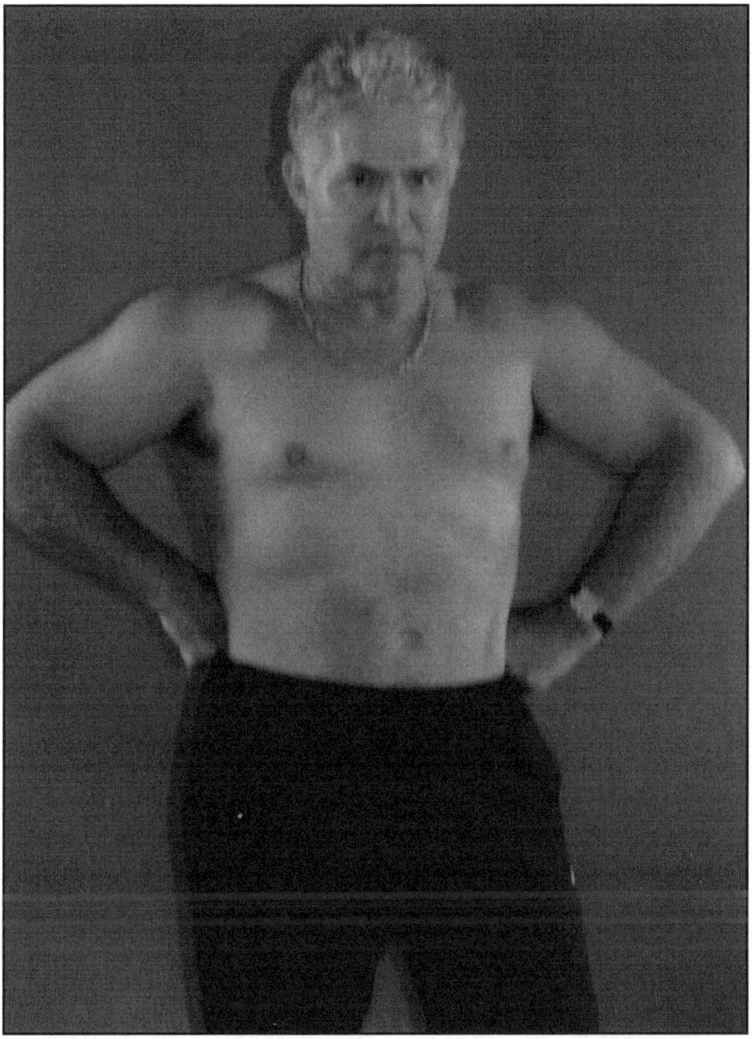

Dr. Carlos Soria 35 years later, after injection of 1500 c.c. of permanent filler into shoulders, arms, and pectoral muscles

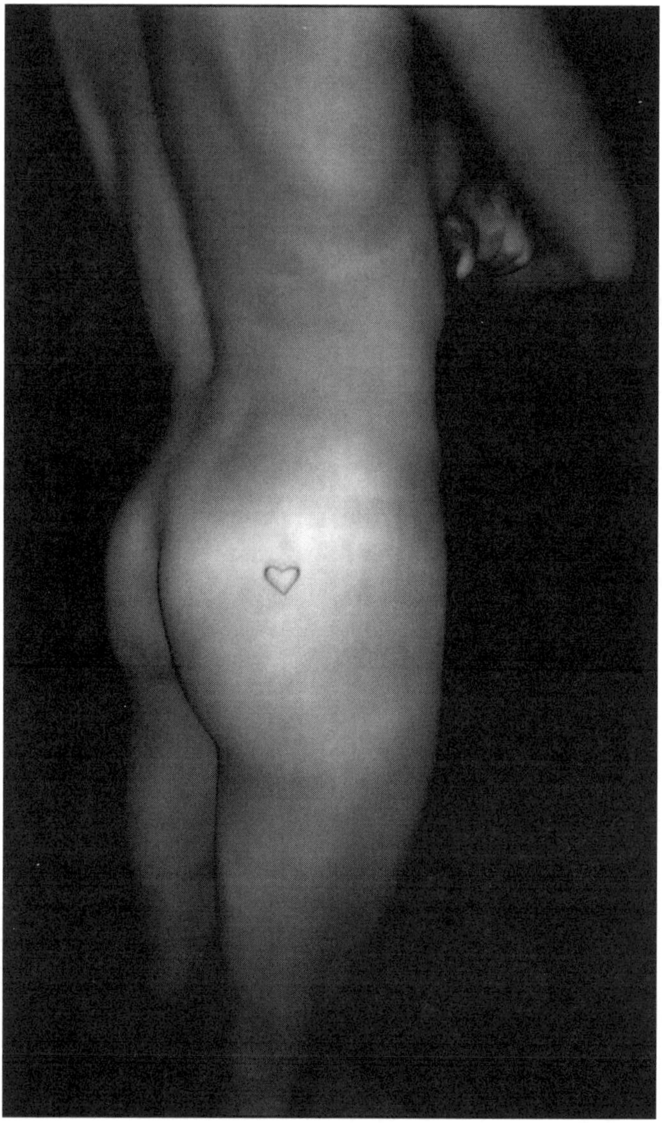

Before gluteal treatment

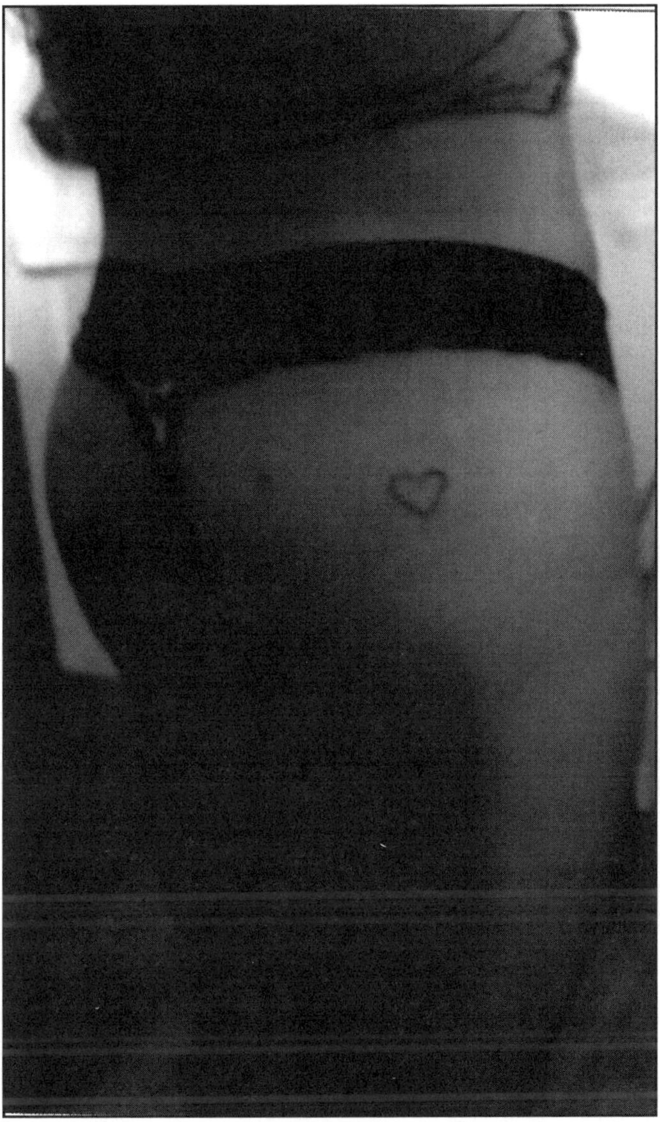

Three months after injection of 160 c.c. of permanent filler in each gluteal muscle

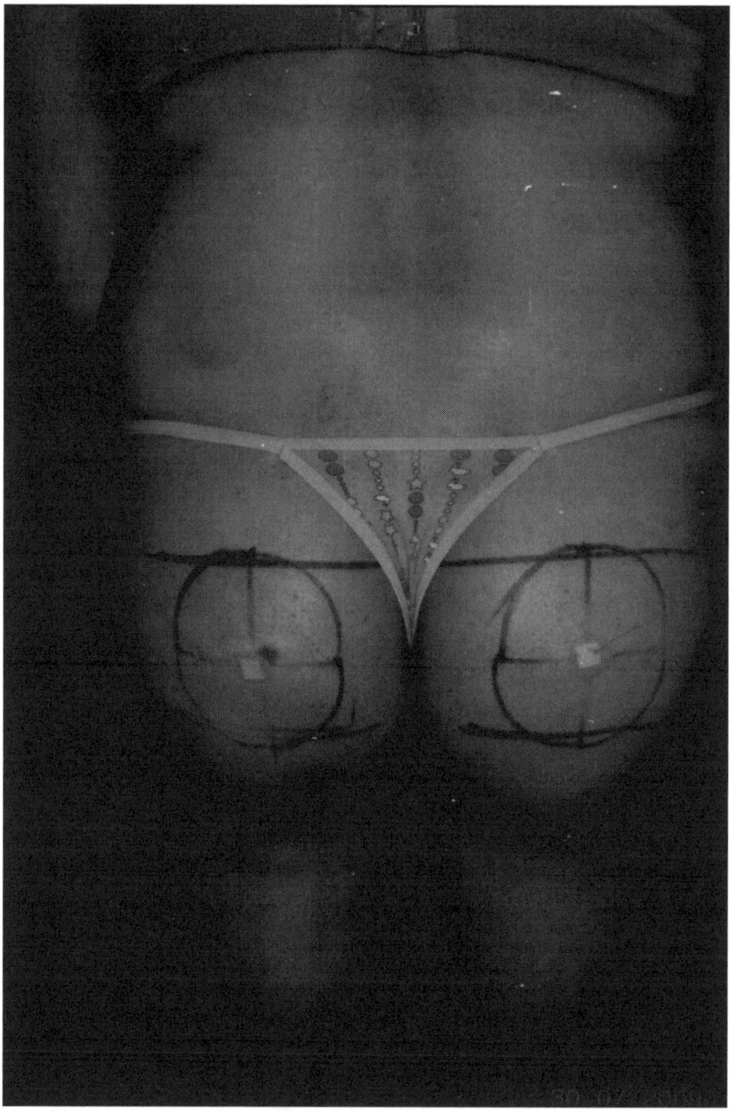

Before

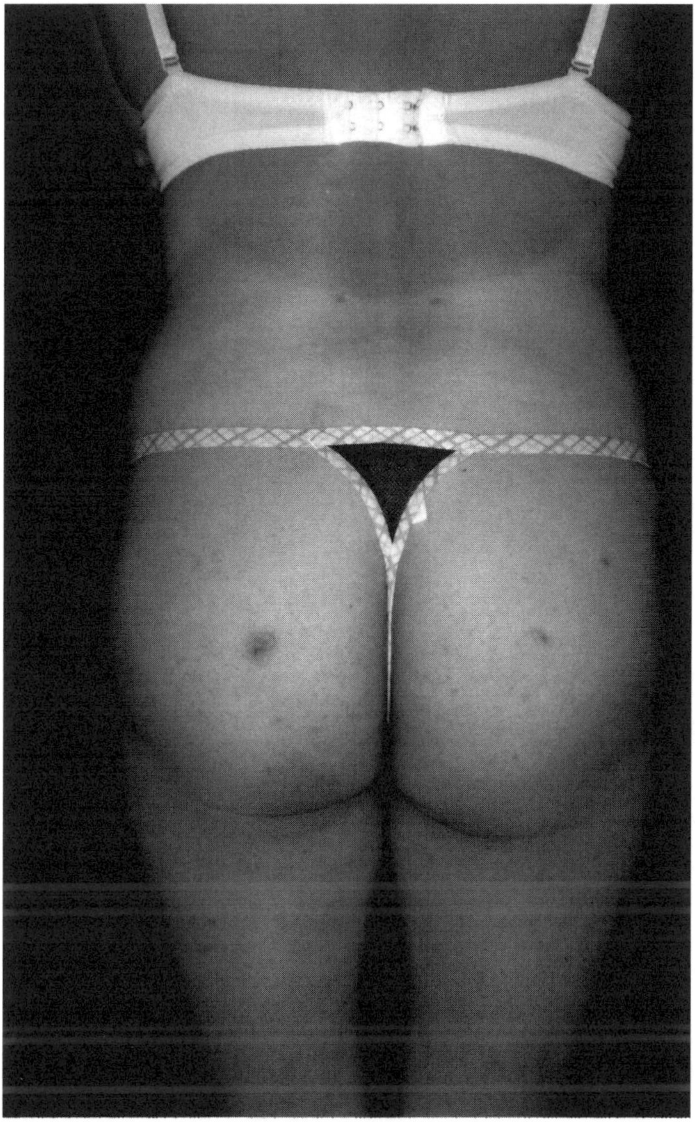

After liposuction and injection of 200 c.c. of permanent filler into each buttock.

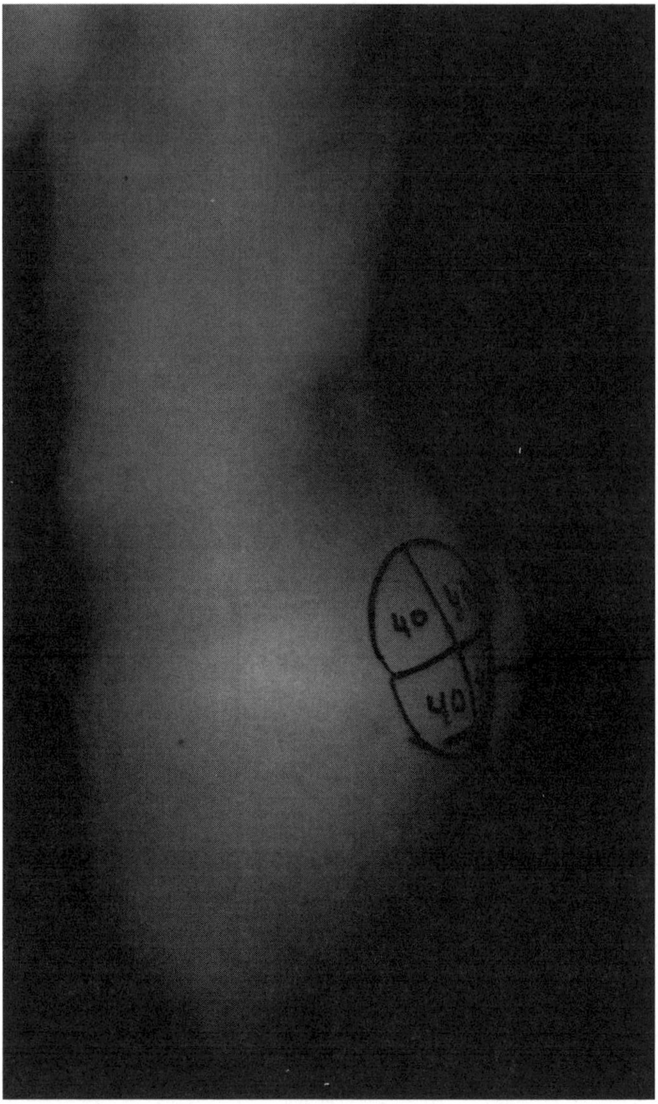

Before

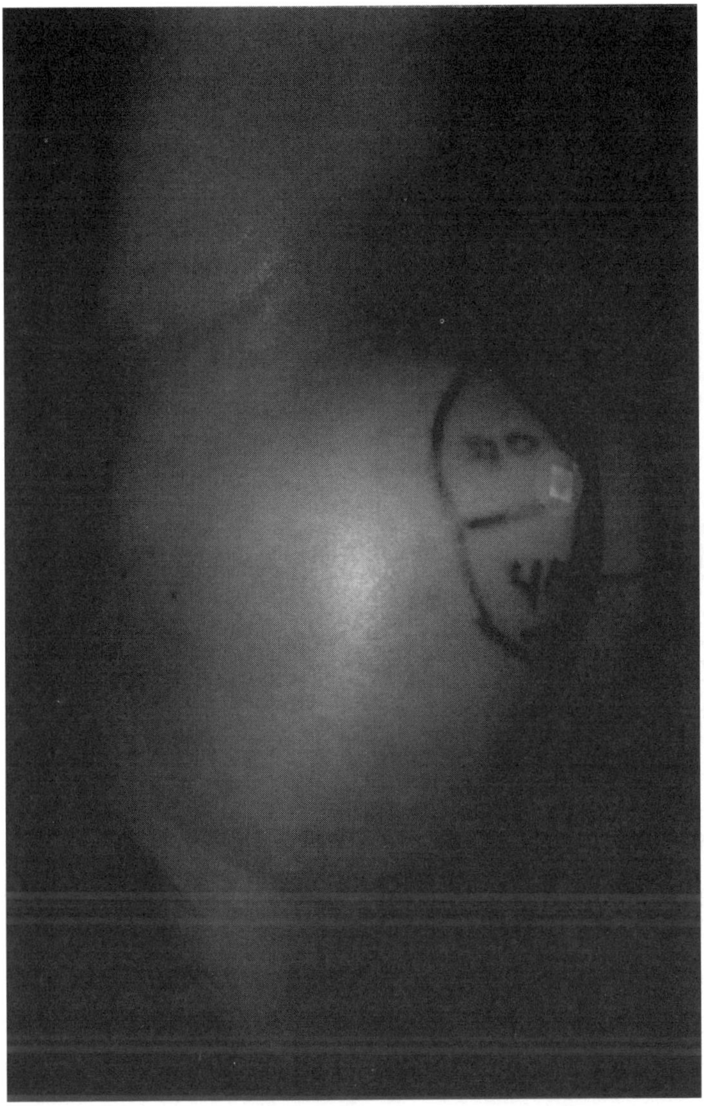

Immediately after injection of 160 c.c. of permanent filler into each buttock

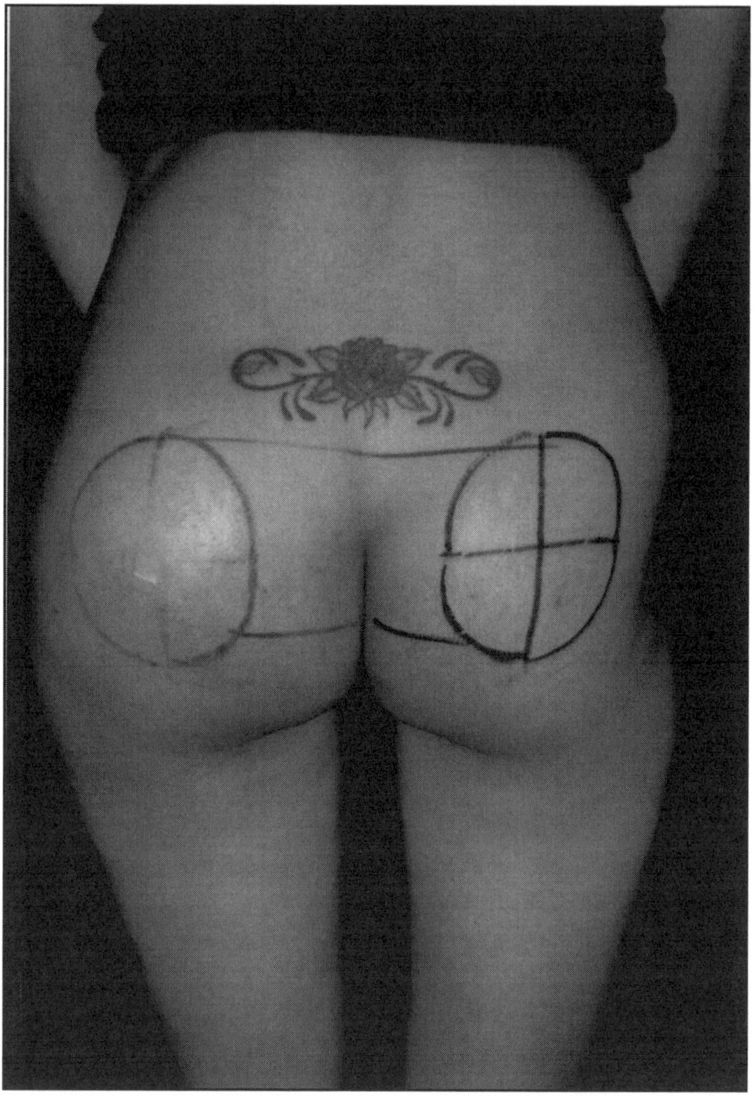

Right side of photo: 25 year old patient before treatment.
Left side of photo: After intramuscular augmentation with
250 c.c. of permanent filler

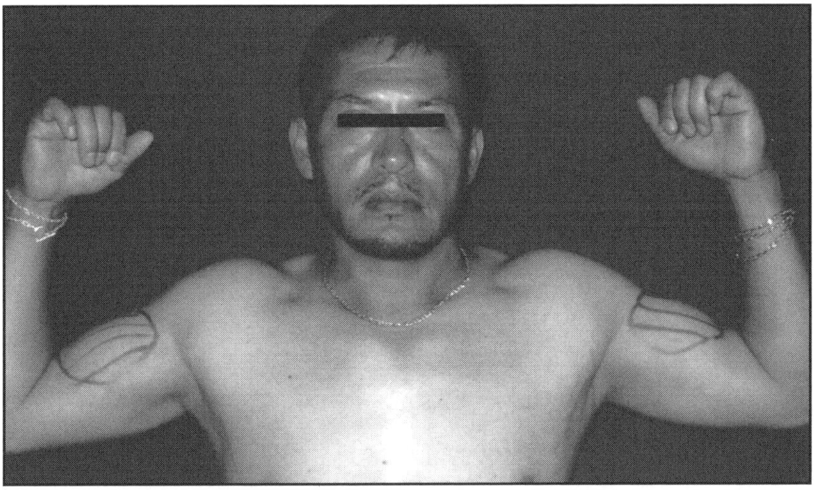

Before biceps augmentation.

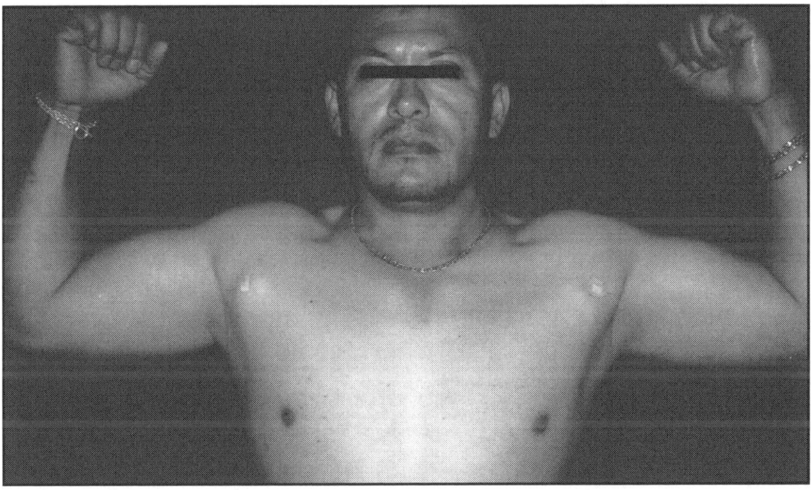

After injection of permanent filler into pectoral and biceps muscles

Further Reading

Andrews JM. Biomaterials em Cirurgia Lastica. In: Melega JM, Aznini AS, Psillakis JM. *Cirurgia Plastica Reparadora e Estetica.* Rio de Janeiro: Medsi, 1992, p. 115.21.

Daane SP. Implantes aloplasticos in: Weinzweig J. *Segrdos em cirurgia platica*. Sao Paulo: Artes Medicas, 2001, p. 61-8.

Ersek RA, Gregory SR, Salisvbury AV. Bioplastique at 6 yars: Clinical Outcome Studies. *Plast Reconstr Surg* 1997; 100:1570-74.

Ersek RA, Stovall RB, Salisbuty AV. Chin augmerntation using minimally invasive technique and bioplastique. *Plast Reconstr Surg* 1994; 95:985-92.

Glemon RA, Young R, Dukat M, Cheng Y. Initial charaterization of PMMA as a discriminative stimulus. *Pharmacal Biochem Behav* 1997 57:151-8.

Guerra M. Injectable fillers (online). [Cited 25 February 2004]. Available from World Wide Web: <http://www.yestheyrefake.net>

Hexsel DM, Hexsel CL, Iyengar V. Liquid injectable silicone: history, mechanism of action, indications, technique, and complications. Semin Cutan Med Surg 2003; 22"1-7-114.

Hoffmann C, Petrovic SS, Soyer P, Kerl H. Adverse Reactions after Cosmetic Lip Augmentation with Permanent Inert Biological Implant Materials. *Am Acad Dermatol*. 1999; 40:100-102.

Kawachi EY, Bertran CA, Reis RR, Alves OL. Bioceramicas: tendenciase perspectivas de uma area interdisciplinar. *Quim Nova* 2000; 23:518-22.

Kenefic NJ, Vaizey CJ, Malouf AJ, Norton CS, Marshall M, Kamm MA. Injectable Silicone Biomaterial for Fcecal Incontinence due to Internal Anal Sphincter Disfunction. Gut 2002; 51:225-8.

Lemperle G, Morhenn V, Chanier U. Human histology and persistence of various injectable filler substances for soft tissue augmentation. *Aesthetic Plast Surg* [online]2004 [Cited 26 February 2004]. Available from World Wide Web <http://pubmed.com>

Nacul AM, Nacul Ap, Greca de Born. A Bioplastique as a complement in conventional plastic surgery. *Aesthetic Plast Surg* 1998; 22:444-50.

Newfill; injetavel Responsavel tecnico Priscila Arruda Bruno. Sao Paulo: Magistral Laboratorio de Manipulac; ao Ltda 2002.

Niechajev I. Lip Enhancement: Surgical Alternatives and Histologic Aspects. *Plast Reconstr Surg* 2000; 105:1173-83.

Orefice RL, Hench LL, Anthony AB. In vitro bioactivity of polymer matrices reinforced with a bioactive glass phase.)

Ousterhout DK, Stelnicki Ej. Plastic Surgery's Plastics. C in *Plast Surg* 1996; 23:183-90.

Rokade AV, Mathews J, Reddy KTV. Tissue Augmentatio Using Bioplastque as a Treatment of Leakage around a Provox 2 Voice Prosthesis *Larnygol Oto* 2003; 117:80-2.

Rudolph CM, Soyer P Petrovic SS, Kerl H. Foreign Body Granulomas Due to Injectable Aesthetic Microimplants. *Am Surg Pathol* 1999; 23:113-7.

Sclafani AP, Romo T 3rd, Parker A, McCormick SA, Cocker R, Jocomo A. Human collagen dispersion (dermalogen) as a dermal filler; persistence and histology compared with bovine collagen. *Ann Plast Surg* 2002; 49:181-8.

Terini E, Sofonio MV. Facial Contouring with Alloplastic implants. In: Aston S, Beasley RW, Thorne CM, Bragg and Smith's Plastic Surgery. New York, Lippincott-Raven, 1997, p. 699-703.

Glossary

Actinia	Protein in muscle fiber (myosin) joins to form the actinomiosina.
Aesthetic	Belonging or relating to the perception or appreciation of beauty.
Analgesic	Pain relieving medicine or drugs that produce analgesia.
Anesthesia	Induced and reversible state of amnesia, analgesia, loss of responsiveness, loss of skeletal muscle reflexes, or decreased fight-or-flight response, or all of these simultaneously.
Antibiotic	A substance produced from certain fungi, bacteria or other organisms that can destroy or inhibit the growth of other microorganisms.
Asymmetry	Not identical on both sides.

Atrophied	Reduce the development or the volume of an organ or other body part for lack of food or exercise.
Augment	To increase in size, such as breast, chin, lips or cheek.
Bactericide	It applies to the substance that destroys bacteria.
Biomaterials	Material tolerated by the body, used for prosthese and other purposes.
Botulinum	A form of food poisoning that usually starts with blurred vision.
Bovine	Pertaining to bulls or cows, a commercial source of collagen.
Cannula	A small tube used in medicine to drain or introduce fluids into the body; the tip of the syringe where the needle is placed.
Cartilage	Flexible skeletal tissue of vertebrates and invertebrates. Formed by isolated groups of cells in a matrix of collagen.
Cellulite	Fat, often referred to as "cottage cheese" in appearance.
Chemical Peel	A procedure used to decrease fine, superficial wrinkles through the use of chemicals.
Chemo-abrasion	A procedure used to correct sking irregularities using combined techniques of chemical application and dermabrasion.

Collagens	Belonging or related to a fibrous protein of connective tissue of the cartilage and bone, transformed into gelatin by cooking.
Comedones	Grain that forms in the skin of the face due to the obstructgion of the excretory duct of a sebaceous gland.
Configuration	Is the set of data and information that characterizes the different elements.
Connective	Ligand linking parts of a single devide or system.
Decrease	Make smaller.
Degeneration	Alteration in body tissues; progressive loss of normal physic and moral.
Dermabrasion	A procedure used to remove the superficial layers of skin using a sanding technique. Used to treat acne scarring and wrinkles around the mouth.
Dermis	Conjunctiva layer that forms part of the skin of vertebrates thicker than the epidermis and below this.
Desquamation	Dry skin shedding in the form of flakes.
Diabetes	A disease in which the body cannot control the amount of sugar in the blood.
Dimorphism	Phenomenon in which there are two ways in its external morphology in a particular species.

Dorsum	The back or outer surface of an organ or part.
Dysplastic	A small line in the skin caused by old age.
Elastic	That of a body, which can more or less completely regain its form and extensions as soon as it stops the action that altered.
Epidermis	This is a concept in anatomy that refers to the ectodermic epithelium that surrounds the body of animals.
Excision	Removal.
Facial	Whitish conjunctiva, which involves different structures.
Fascia	A band of connective tissue supporting or binding together internal organs or parts of the body,
Fat	Butter or animal tallow.
Fibroblast	Connective tissue cell, secreting and cross-linked elastin, which form interstitial fibers.
Frown lines	Deep wrinkles on the forehead between the eyebrows.
Hyperpigmentation	Increased pigmentation or color, Hyperpigmented skin is abnormally dark. Hyperpigmentation occurs when an excess amount of melatonin is produced.
Hypertension	A medical term for unusually high blood pressure.

Implants	Device, prosthetic or substance that is placed on the body to improve some of its functions, or for an aesthetic purpose.
Inert	Non-irritating to the body.
Laser	An acronym for Light Amplification Stimulated Emission of Radiation.
Lateral	Situated next to something.
Lethargic	Lacking in energy; feeling unwilling or unable to do anything.
Laxity	Looseness.
LIS	Liquid Injectible Silicon technique.
Malar	Cheek area.
Nasal	Pertaining to the nose.
Nasolabial	Deep wrinkles located between the upper lip and nose.
Obesity	Extremely fat.
Oxidize	If a substance oxidizes, it combines with oxygen and loses hydrogen to form another substance; if something oxidizes a substance, it causes it to do this. Action an effect of rust or corrosion.
Papillary dermis	One of the elements that make up the dermis; It is the most superficial layer and consists primarily of connective tissue.

Peeling	A cosmetic dermatology practice that is widely used today. The success of the treatment depends on the knowledge of the practitioner, the guidelines for application, and professional training.
Perioral rhytids	Deep wrinkles found around the mouth.
Pigmentation	Normal coloration of the skin or tissue that can be caused by various reasons. Age and the sun are the most common,
Pliability	Able to bend easily.
Postoperative	The period occurring immediately after a surgical operation.
Prophylactic	It serves to introduce or protect against disease.
Protein	A substance or organic compound of high molecular weight and complete structure, formed by the union of numerous aminoacids through peptide bonds.
Prosthesis	An artificial part, such as a breast implant, inserted into or attached to the body.
Ptosis	Drooping, such as breasts or eyelids.
Reticular dermis	One of the many elements of the skin. It is the lowest layer and the thicker dermis, the thickness varies in different parts.
Rhytidosis	Excessive folds of skin, or wrinkles.

Rounding	Round shape to something.
Seculorum	The belief that religion should not be involved with the ordinary social and political activities of a country.
Septum	Central wall dividing the nasal passages.
Suture	Sewing to close a wound's edges.
Toxin	Poisonous substance produced by the metabolic actiity of certain organisms; toxins are listed by the action of microorganisms.
Vascular	Whole and irrigation of small, you blood and lymph vessels in a tissue, organ or body region.
Vital signs	Measurements of various physiological statistics often taken by health professionals to assess the most basic bodily functions. Vital signs are an essential part of the representation of the case.
Wrinkles	Small lines in the skin caused by old age.

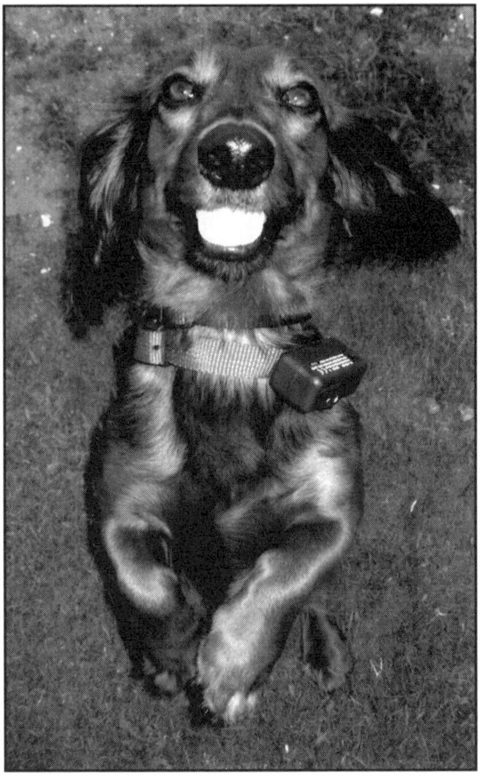

Daddy, Daddy, I just bit another patient —
I hope you have insurance!
(Dr. Soria's dog, Chicha.)

About the Author

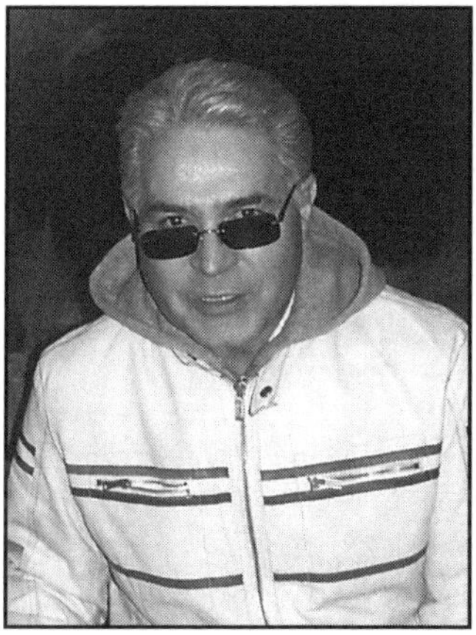

Dr. Carlos Soria has spent more than 35 years in the medical profession, completing the necessary education and training to become not only an M.D. but also a Ph.D. His initial M.D. degree was obtained at the University of Mexico City. He also received a grant to study at the London University for five more years, achieving a diploma in Physical Medicine, a diploma of Clinical Rheumatology and in the research field, and a Ph.D. in Pharmacology. When he returned to Mexico City, Dr. Soria worked as a teacher of Pharmacology at the School of Medicine and as a consultant in Rheumatology for the National Institute of Cardiology. After the above mentioned posts, he moved to Tijuana, Baja California, Mexico and worked as a full time professor at the Medical and Dental schools.

As a private physician, he founded the "Villa of Youth" a European Skin Rejuvenation and Plastic Surgery center in Rosarito, Baja Mexico. With a team of specialists Dr. Soria has treated hundreds of American patients that feel the quality of medicine in Baja California, Mexico, is as good as in U.S.A. and the prices are far more competitive. Dr. Soria is married to an English lady, Gaynor, and has 3 children, one of whom is an M.D. who has worked beside him for the last 10+ years at the Villa of Youth.

Dr. Soria has traveled the world teaching his medical procedures and training many doctors in the field of "medical aesthetics and non-surgical procedures."

After nearly four decades of medical practice, he has written this book to share his experiences and techniques with other doctors as well as to educate patients that are considering their options for "Beauty without the Scalpel."

Dr. Carlos Soria and his team are willing to train doctors in the field of non-invasive medical aesthetic procedures.

Please contact us at:
Dr. Carlos Soria, M.D., Ph.D.
Villa of Youth
P. O. Box 433856
San Diego, CA 92143

www.villaofyouth.com
drsoria@villaofyouth.com
(619) 892-2157
(888) 901-2744

ANNOUNCING the new Villa of Youth Ocean Project

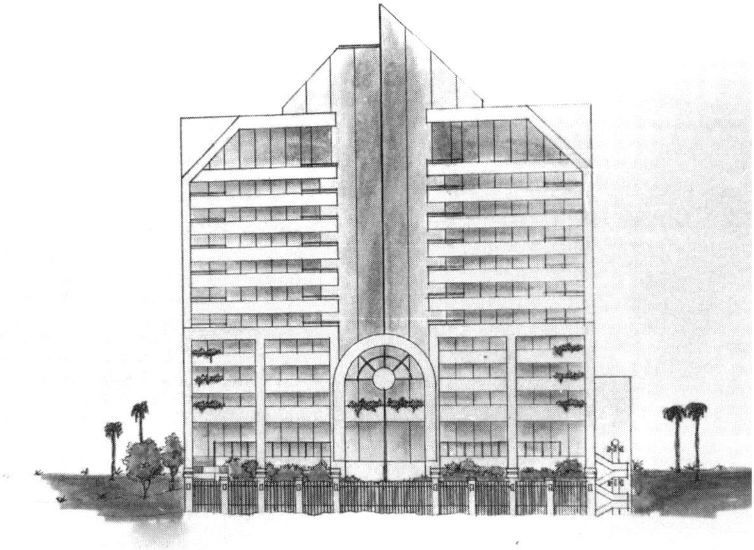

A property of 2100 meters adjacent to the state beach in Playas de Tijuana has been purchased. Plans are in the offing for a 12-floor complex with underground parking, a restaurant, conference rooms, a swimming pool-jacuzzi, and direct access to the beach. There will be a clinic, an assisted living facility, an entertainment and physical therapy complex, and 8 levels of condominiums (a total of 32 condominiums). The clinic will be our flagship, with treatment plans available for 1 week, 12 days, 1 month, and 3 months. We will also offer stem cell therapies that are only available in a limited number of locations.

The clinic will offer:

- Leading edge diagnosis
- Retardation of aging
- Revitalization (internal)
- Rejuvenation (external): plastic and nonplastic surgery

Condominium features:

- 100 square meters
- 3 bedrooms, 2-1/2 bathrooms
- Ocean view from each condo
- Fully gated community

Assisted living facility features:

- Private room for each patient
- 24/7 bilingual staff, medical personnel, and ambulance service
- Gymnasium with daily physiotherapy and exercise classes
- Fully-staffed kitchen; special diets available
- Full housekeeping service
- Complimentary transportation to their American doctor
- On-site dentist and psychologist
- Library
- Chapel

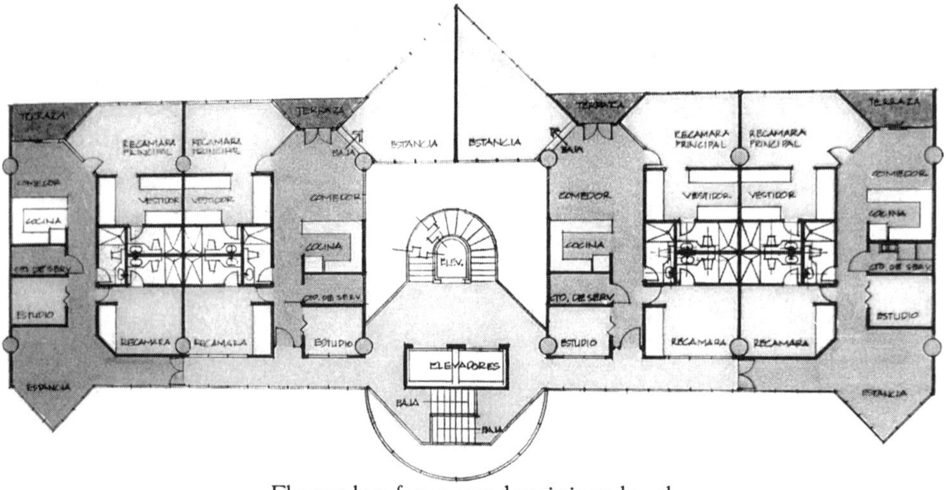

Floor plan for a condominium level

How Can You Participate?

The income for this project will come from two sources:

- To start the program we will sell 100 shares for $20,000 dollars each, which will represent a total of 49% interest in the business.
- The remaining income will come from the sale of the 32 condominiums.

The original investors of 100 shares will have a profit of 49% of the sales from the condominiums, as well as a 10% permanent income from the medical Assisted Living Program and VIP executive service at 50% discount.

The investors in the condominiums can rent their units to the patients from the clinic. Additionally, if they recommend the services of the clinic to their friends and customers they will receive the rental fees of their units as well as a 10% commission for the referral. That way we will have 32 permanent investors/promoters.

For more information on investment opportunities, please contact Dr. Carlos Soria:

By phone: 888-901-2744
By email: drsoria@villaofyouth.com

Please watch for the second book in the series:

Permanent Body Augmentation Without the Scalpel